Advances in
IMMUNOLOGY

VOLUME **113**

Immunity to *Listeria monocytogenes*

Advances in IMMUNOLOGY

VOLUME 113

Immunity to *Listeria monocytogenes*

Edited by

EMIL R. UNANUE

Department of Pathology and Immunology, Washington University School of Medicine, St. Louis, Missouri, USA

JAVIER A. CARRERO

Department of Pathology and Immunology, Washington University School of Medicine, St. Louis, Missouri, USA

ELSEVIER

AMSTERDAM • BOSTON • HEIDELBERG • LONDON
NEW YORK • OXFORD • PARIS • SAN DIEGO
SAN FRANCISCO • SINGAPORE • SYDNEY • TOKYO
Academic Press is an imprint of Elsevier

Academic Press is an imprint of Elsevier
525 B Street, Suite 1900, San Diego, CA 92101-4495, USA
225 Wyman Street, Waltham, MA 02451, USA
32 Jamestown Road, London, NW1 7BY, UK
Radarweg 29, PO Box 211, 1000 AE Amsterdam, The Netherlands

First edition 2012

ISBN: 978-0-12-394590-7
ISSN: 0065-2776

For information on all Academic Press publications
visit our website at elsevierdirect.com

Printed and bound by CPI Group (UK) Ltd, Croydon, CR0 4YY

Transferred to Digital Print 2012

CONTENTS

CONTRIBUTORS

Numbers in parentheses indicate the pages on which the authors' contributions begin.

Kristina A. Archer
Department of Molecular and Cell Biology, University of California, Berkeley, Berkeley, California, USA (*135*)

Vladimir P. Badovinac
Department of Pathology; Interdisciplinary Graduate Program in Immunology, University of Iowa, Iowa City, Iowa, USA (*51*)

John H. Brumell
Cell Biology Program, Hospital for Sick Children; Institute of Medical Science; and Department of Molecular Genetics University of Toronto, Toronto, Ontario, Canada (*7*)

Javier A. Carrero
Department of Pathology and Immunology, Washington University School of Medicine, St. Louis, Missouri, USA (*1, 157*)

Stephanie A. Condotta
Department of Pathology, University of Iowa, Iowa City, Iowa, USA (*51*)

Pascale Cossart
Institut Pasteur, Unité des Interactions Bactéries-Cellules; Inserm U604; and INRA, USC2020, Paris, France (*19*)

Mark A. Czuczman
Cell Biology Program, Hospital for Sick Children; Department of Molecular Genetics, University of Toronto, Toronto, Ontario, Canada (*7*)

Brian T. Edelson
Department of Pathology and Immunology, Washington University School of Medicine, St. Louis, Missouri, USA (*33*)

Patrick Guirnalda
Department of Microbiology, Perelman School of Medicine, University of Pennsylvania, Philadelphia, Pennsylvania, USA (*81*)

John T. Harty
Department of Pathology; Department of Microbiology; Interdisciplinary Graduate Program in Immunology, University of Iowa, Iowa City, Iowa, USA (*51*)

Darren E. Higgins
Department of Microbiology and Immunobiology, Harvard Medical School, Boston, Massachusetts, USA (*7*)

Grace Y. Lam
Cell Biology Program, Hospital for Sick Children; Institute of Medical Science, University of Toronto, Toronto, Ontario, Canada (*7*)

Serge Mostowy
Institut Pasteur, Unité des Interactions Bactéries-Cellules; Inserm U604; and INRA, USC2020, Paris, France (*19*)

Eric G. Pamer
Infectious Diseases Service, Department of Medicine, Immunology Program, Sloan-Kettering Institute, Memorial Sloan-Kettering Cancer Center, New York, USA (*119*)

Yvonne Paterson
Department of Microbiology, Perelman School of Medicine, University of Pennsylvania, Philadelphia, Pennsylvania, USA (*81*)

Daniel A. Portnoy
Graduate Group in Microbiology; Department of Molecular and Cell Biology; and School of Public Health, University of California, Berkeley, Berkeley, California, USA (*135*)

Chris S. Rae
Department of Molecular and Cell Biology, University of California, Berkeley, Berkeley, California, USA (*135*)

Martin J. Richer
Department of Microbiology, University of Iowa, Iowa City, Iowa, USA (*51*)

John-Demian Sauer
Department of Medical Microbiology and Immunology, University of Wisconsin-Madison, Madison, Wisconsin, USA (*135*)

Natalya V. Serbina
Infectious Diseases Service, Department of Medicine, Immunology Program, Sloan-Kettering Institute, Memorial Sloan-Kettering Cancer Center, New York, USA (*119*)

Chao Shi
Infectious Diseases Service, Department of Medicine, Immunology Program, Sloan-Kettering Institute, Memorial Sloan-Kettering Cancer Center, New York, USA (*119*)

Emil R. Unanue
Department of Pathology and Immunology, Washington University School of Medicine, St. Louis, Missouri, USA (*1, 157*)

Chelsea E. Witte
Graduate Group in Microbiology, University of California, Berkeley, Berkeley, California, USA (*135*)

Laurence Wood
Department of Microbiology, Perelman School of Medicine, University of Pennsylvania, Philadelphia, Pennsylvania, USA (*81*)

Joshua J. Woodward
Department of Microbiology, University of Washington, Seattle, Washington, USA (*135*)

CHAPTER 1

Studies with *Listeria Monocytogenes* Lead the Way

Emil R. Unanue and **Javier A. Carrero**

One of us (E. R. U.) last edited an issue reviewing *Listeria monocytogenes* in 1997 (Unanue, 1997a,b). Many of us thought that many aspects of this infection had been examined and that more progress was going to be limited. It soon became clear that this was not the case and that this fascinating bacterium was going to keep microbiologists, cell biologists, and immunologists busy for some time.

L. monocytogenes, a Gram-positive facultative intracellular pathogen, has a limited infectivity and is not one of the major bacterial pathogens. In the United States of America, the number of documented infections is low (~1600 cases annually), although mortality is high particularly in immunodeficient individuals (~200 deaths annually). The impetus for the many investigations on *L. monocytogenes* lies in its fascinating life history. The tricks that *L. monocytogenes* uses have helped us learn many fundamental principles of immunology, pathogenesis, and cellular biology. Infection starts by invasion of epithelial surfaces through a series of well-defined invasins that target species-specific host cell-surface receptors (Gaillard *et al.*, 1991). These interactions are not optimal in the mouse, so infection through the natural oral route is inefficient (Lecuit *et al.*, 2001). Experimentally this limitation is avoided by infecting systemically through either intraperitoneal or intravenous routes. Following systemic infection, bacteria are quickly phagocytosed by macrophages and neutrophils. The bacteria are well adapted to this lifestyle and quickly exit the phagosome and swim inside the cytosol of infected cells by polymerizing actin (Tilney and

Department of Pathology and Immunology, Washington University School of Medicine, St. Louis, Missouri, USA

Advances in Immunology, Volume 113
ISSN 0065-2776, DOI: 10.1016/B978-0-12-394590-7.00009-9

Portnoy, 1989). Adaptive immunity involving T cells follows, leading to complete clearance of the bacteria (Lane and Unanue, 1972).

In the 1997 introduction, a point was made of the seminal findings in experimental tuberculosis that gave much guidance to the field of host resistance to intracellular pathogens: the discovery of the tuberculin reaction by Robert Koch and the definition of delayed hypersensitivity; the identification of the tuberculous granulomas and of the activated macrophages; the seminal finding that lymphocytes and not antibody transferred protection; the discovery of cytokines. All these pointed to a mechanism of protection very different from those to extracellular bacteria in which antibodies and complement were the major control molecules. *L. monocytogenes* comes into the picture following Mackaness' establishment of the basic parameters for infection in mice (Mackaness, 1962). This led to a critical examination of the mechanisms of resistance, confirming an early observation that serum from infected animals did not transfer protection (Osebold and Sawyer, 1957). Acquired immunity to *L. monocytogenes* was transferred only by live cells (Miki and Mackaness, 1964) (References cited here are not comprehensive; for a detailed list, refer to recent reviews (Pamer, 2004; Stavru *et al.*, 2011)). This was the impetus in trying to figure out by which process *L. monocytogenes* resistance was accomplished.

Mackaness' studies led the way and soon *L. monocytogenes* became the favorite intracellular pathogen to study. It was an easy microbe to examine, of low pathogenicity to humans so it could be handled in regular laboratories, and the mouse was an ideal host and highly susceptible to systemic delivery (in contrast to *Mycobacterium tuberculosis*). Studying listeriosis may provide insights into granulomatous inflammation and allow a better understanding of tuberculosis was one way of thinking. After years of analysis, the investigations of *L. monocytogenes* led to major understanding of bacterial pathogenesis and antibacterial immunological reactions. Some basic issues were particularly common between infections (listeriosis and tuberculosis); T cell participation, lack of protection by antibodies, cytokine responses, granulomas are some of them. However the differences between both infections are striking, there is sterilizing immunity in listeriosis; in tuberculosis, we find latency and persistent occult infection.

For immunologists, it became the ideal organism for many reasons: the mouse allowed examination of different cellular components using the wealth of reagents available to track and examine cells and cytokines. Importantly, resistance involved a number of overlapping stages each under the influence of particular sets of cells and cytokines (Unanue, 1997a). One can distinguish the early stage, now named as the "innate" immunity stage, and the specific T cells stage that follows and that results in sterilizing immunity. It was the analysis of *L. monocytogenes* that defined and characterized each stage and then set the basis for examining other infections. One can say that everyone's favorite cell or cytokine participates to some extent or another in this infection.

Examining the innate phase allowed the cellular rules for antigen processing to be established (Ziegler and Unanue, 1981). This was the first bacterial infection in which Major Histocompatibility (MHC) restriction was documented (Zinkernagel, 1974). The role of neutrophils was identified the first time that it was conclusively proven that these cells, well known to be essential for the control of extracellular bacteria, were also vital for control of an intracellular bacteria (Conlan and North, 1991). The important role for cytokines was highlighted in *L. monocytogenes,* the first infection in which it was conclusively established that interferon-gamma was the key protective cytokine. Indeed, the first neutralizing anticytokines monoclonal antibodies were tested in murine listeriosis (Buchmeier and Schreiber, 1985). Features of the lymphocyte response such as the initial burst, memory, the cooperativity between CD4 and CD8 T cells led to major insights (Busch *et al.*, 1998; North, 1973; Pamer, 2004). Because *L. monocytogenes* infection results in presentation to both CD4 and CD8 T cells, the pathways of presentation have been the subject of study by many (Pamer *et al.*, 1991).

As important and seminal has been the contribution of microbiologists to *L. monocytogenes* pathogenesis. Having the genome entirely decoded in Pascale Cossart's laboratory became a breakthrough leading into the biological context of various bacterial proteins (Glaser *et al.*, 2001). The property of *L. monocytogenes,* in having an intracellular phase in the cytosol of the infected cell, is exceptional (Tilney and Portnoy, 1989). This cytosolic stage is not found in most bacterial infections (Portnoy *et al.*, 1988) and became a focus of studies on the mechanisms for entry into the cytosol, on the proteins that are relevant for entry, on the way that the bacteria moves, and of the consequences of such entry (reviewed by Dussurget *et al.*, 2004). This localization in the cytosol not only provides *L. monocytogenes* a means to evade the host response but also results in the activation of a number of signaling pathways (O'Riordan *et al.*, 2002). It also involves the presentation of epitopes by class I MHC molecules (Brunt *et al.*, 1990).

There are few microbes in which mechanisms of attachment to leukocytes and epithelial cells has been so well studied as in listeriosis to the extent that binding paradigms have been established (Bonazzi *et al.*, 2009). One area lagging behind in listeriosis concerns the natural portal of infection, the gastrointestinal tract (Lecuit *et al.*, 2001). Most studies cited above have used the intravenous or intraperitoneal infection resulting mostly in liver and spleen infections. The examination of the biology of the gastrointestinal tract is moving at an accelerated pace and forthcoming will be the studies on listeriosis.

L. monocytogenes produces a cytolysin, listeriolysin O (LLO), with many unique properties that have called the attention not only of microbiologists and immunologists but also of biochemists and structural biologists (Schnupf and Portnoy, 2007; Tweten *et al.*, 2001). LLO is the major factor responsible for virulence, the major molecule allowing access of the microbe to the cytosol, and a major immunogen that contributes epitopes to both the CD4 and CD8 pathways of presentation.

We have assembled here a number of recent contributors to this field. John Brumell reviews autophagy during *L. monocytogenes* infection. Interestingly, the bacteria avoid autophagy-mediated killing to allow survival in both the cytosol and in modified vacuoles. Pascale Cossart examines various virulence strategies of *L. monocytogenes*, including new discovered host histone modifications. These are findings that have been first made during *Listeria* infection, and it will be interesting to determine how microbes exploit these insults to their hosts. Brian Edelson reviews the important issue of localization of *L. monocytogenes* in infected organs, particularly the spleen. Here is another example on how this bacterium has added new surprising insights, particularly on the role of one subset of dendritic cells, the $CD11c^{+}$/ $CD8\alpha^{+}$ set. John Harty and colleagues investigate the development of CD8 memory responses against *L. monocytogenes* and show us how much has been learned about memory from this one bacterial infection. Eric Pamer and colleagues summarize the work on the role of $Ly6c^{hi}$ monocytes in the control of listeriosis. This is an important phase because it recruits new innate effectors to counter *L. monocytogenes* infection when it is at its peak. Exploiting *L. monocytogenes* to make better vaccines against other pathogens or tumors is promising field. Yvonne Paterson covers the approaches that have been used to adapt *L. monocytogenes* and its products to immunize against tumors. Daniel Portnoy and associates review new insights into the cytosolic activities of *L. monocytogenes*. This includes conserved microbial products that are sensed by the host to initiate the immune response. Finally, we review our studies on lymphocyte apoptosis and the role of type I interferons. Listeriosis has a phase of early lymphocyte apoptosis that is obligatory and contributes heavily to the infection.

We thank our colleagues who joined us with their contributions and await the next review perhaps much sooner than before, seeing how the research in listeriosis continues to grow.

REFERENCES

Bonazzi, M., Lecuit, M., and Cossart, P. (2009). *Listeria monocytogenes* internalin and E-cadherin: From structure to pathogenesis. *Cell. Microbiol.* **11,** 693–702.

Brunt, L. M., Portnoy, D. A., and Unanue, E. R. (1990). Presentation of *Listeria monocytogenes* to CD8+ T cells requires secretion of hemolysin and intracellular bacterial growth. *J. Immunol.* **145,** 3540–3546.

Buchmeier, N. A., and Schreiber, R. D. (1985). Requirement of endogenous interferon-gamma production for resolution of *Listeria monocytogenes* infection. *Proc. Natl. Acad. Sci. USA* **82,** 7404–7408.

Busch, D. H., Pilip, I. M., Vijh, S., and Pamer, E. G. (1998). Coordinate regulation of complex T cell populations responding to bacterial infection. *Immunity* **8,** 353–362.

Conlan, J. W., and North, R. J. (1991). Neutrophil-mediated dissolution of infected host cells as a defense strategy against a facultative intracellular bacterium. *J. Exp. Med.* **174,** 741–744.

Dussurget, O., Pizarro-Cerda, J., and Cossart, P. (2004). Molecular determinants of *Listeria monocytogenes* virulence. *Annu. Rev. Microbiol.* **58,** 587–610.

Gaillard, J. L., Berche, P., Frehel, C., Gouin, E., and Cossart, P. (1991). Entry of *L. monocytogenes* into cells is mediated by internalin, a repeat protein reminiscent of surface antigens from gram-positive cocci. *Cell* **65,** 1127–1141.

Glaser, P., Frangeul, L., Buchrieser, C., Rusniok, C., Amend, A., Baquero, F., Berche, P., Bloecker, H., Brandt, P., Chakraborty, T., Charbit, A., and Chetouani, F. (2001). Comparative genomics of *Listeria* species. *Science* **294,** 849–852.

Lane, F. C., and Unanue, E. R. (1972). Requirement of thymus (T) lymphocytes for resistance to listeriosis. *J. Exp. Med.* **135,** 1104–1112.

Lecuit, M., Vandormael-Pournin, S., Lefort, J., Huerre, M., Gounon, P., Dupuy, C., Babinet, C., and Cossart, P. (2001). A transgenic model for listeriosis: Role of internalin in crossing the intestinal barrier. *Science* **292,** 1722–1725.

Mackaness, G. B. (1962). Cellular resistance to infection. *J. Exp. Med.* **116,** 381–406.

Miki, K., and Mackaness, G. B. (1964). The passive transfer of acquired resistance to *Listeria monocytogenes*. *J. Exp. Med.* **120,** 93–103.

North, R. J. (1973). Cellular mediators of anti-*Listeria* immunity as an enlarged population of short lived, replicating T cells. Kinetics of their production. *J. Exp. Med.* **138,** 342–355.

O'Riordan, M., Yi, C. H., Gonzales, R., Lee, K. D., and Portnoy, D. A. (2002). Innate recognition of bacteria by a macrophage cytosolic surveillance pathway. *Proc. Natl. Acad. Sci. USA* **99,** 13861–13866.

Osebold, J. W., and Sawyer, M. T. (1957). Immunization studies on listeriosis in mice. *J. Immunol.* **78,** 262–268.

Pamer, E. G. (2004). Immune responses to *Listeria monocytogenes*. *Nat. Rev. Immunol.* **4,** 812–823.

Pamer, E. G., Harty, J. T., and Bevan, M. J. (1991). Precise prediction of a dominant class I MHC-restricted epitope of *Listeria monocytogenes*. *Nature* **353,** 852–855.

Portnoy, D. A., Jacks, P. S., and Hinrichs, D. J. (1988). Role of hemolysin for the intracellular growth of *Listeria monocytogenes*. *J. Exp. Med.* **167,** 1459–1471.

Schnupf, P., and Portnoy, D. A. (2007). Listeriolysin O: A phagosome-specific lysin. *Microbes Infect.* **9,** 1176–1187.

Stavru, F., Archambaud, C., and Cossart, P. (2011). Cell biology and immunology of *Listeria monocytogenes* infections: Novel insights. *Immunol. Rev.* **240,** 160–184.

Tilney, L. G., and Portnoy, D. A. (1989). Actin filaments and the growth, movement, and spread of the intracellular bacterial parasite, *Listeria monocytogenes*. *J. Cell Biol.* **109,** 1597–1608.

Tweten, R. K., Parker, M. W., and Johnson, A. E. (2001). The cholesterol-dependent cytolysins. *Curr. Top. Microbiol. Immunol.* **257,** 15–33.

Unanue, E. R. (1997a). Studies in listeriosis show the strong symbiosis between the innate cellular system and the T-cell response. *Immunol. Rev.* **158,** 11–25.

Unanue, E. R. (1997b). Why listeriosis? A perspective on cellular immunity to infection. *Immunol. Rev.* **158,** 5–9.

Ziegler, K., and Unanue, E. R. (1981). Identification of a macrophage antigen-processing event required for I-region-restricted antigen presentation to T lymphocytes. *J. Immunol.* **127,** 1869–1875.

Zinkernagel, R. M. (1974). Restriction by H-2 gene complex of transfer of cell-mediated immunity to *Listeria monocytogenes*. *Nature* **251,** 230–233.

CHAPTER 2

Interactions of *Listeria monocytogenes* with the Autophagy System of Host Cells

Grace Y. Lam,[*,†,1] **Mark A. Czuczman,**[*,‡,1] **Darren E. Higgins,**[§] and **John H. Brumell**[*,†,‡]

Contents

Abstract

Macrophages are immune cells that participate in the host defense against bacterial pathogens. These cells mediate bacterial clearance by internalizing bacteria into a phagosome, which ultimately fuses with lysosomes to kill bacteria. One bacterial strategy to evade killing in the phagosome is to escape from this compartment prior to lysosomal fusion. *Listeria monocytogenes* is a classic example of a "cytosol-adapted pathogen" in that it can rapidly escape from the phagosome in macrophages (and other cell types) and replicate rapidly in the cytosol. Phagosome escape also enables cell-to-cell spread by the bacteria through a bacterial driven actin-based

* Cell Biology Program, Hospital for Sick Children, Toronto, Ontario, Canada
† Institute of Medical Science, University of Toronto, Toronto, Ontario, Canada
‡ Department of Molecular Genetics, University of Toronto, Toronto, Ontario, Canada
§ Department of Microbiology and Immunobiology, Harvard Medical School, Boston, Massachusetts, USA
1 These authors contributed equally to this chapter.

Advances in Immunology, Volume 113
ISSN 0065-2776, DOI: 10.1016/B978-0-12-394590-7.00008-7

motility mechanism. How the bacteria escape the phagosome and evade host cellular defenses, including autophagy, will be discussed in this review. We also discuss an underappreciated population of *L. monocytogenes* that can replicate in macrophage vacuoles and how these may be important for the establishment of chronic infections.

1. INTRODUCTION

Listeria monocytogenes is the causative agent of listeriosis, a gastroenteritis that is self-limiting in healthy individuals but may become severe and systemic in immunocompromised individuals, the elderly and pregnant women (Rocourt and Bille, 1997). This Gram-positive, rod-shaped bacterium provides an important paradigm for host–pathogen interactions since it can replicate within a variety of host cell types during infection. This includes macrophages, cells of the innate immune system that are normally capable of killing bacteria. To replicate in macrophages, bacterial pathogens have evolved different mechanisms to avoid delivery to the lysosome upon uptake by host cells (reviewed in Flannagan *et al.*, 2009; Kirkegaard *et al.*, 2004; Kumar and Valdivia, 2009). What has intrigued researchers in the *L. monocytogenes* field is the ability of these bacteria to escape from the phagosome and replicate rapidly in the cytosol of host cells. The bacteria can escape from the phagosome via the activity of three virulence factors: listeriolysin O (LLO) and two phospholipase C enzymes, PI-PLC and PC-PLC. Upon phagosome escape, *L. monocytogenes* can then replicate rapidly in the nutrient rich cytosol. Another virulence factor, ActA, then mediates the nucleation of an actin tail on one end of the bacteria. Polymerization of the actin tail allows the bacteria to "rocket" into neighboring cells, allowing for cell-to-cell spread of the infection (Tilney and Portnoy, 1989). The ability to escape from the phagosome prior to killing in lysosomes ultimately enables *L. monocytogenes* to replicate rapidly in the cytosol and spread to neighboring cells. Below, we will elaborate on the known host and bacterial factors that facilitate phagosome escape by these bacteria.

In addition to phagosomal defenses, *L. monocytogenes* must counter autophagy, which has recently emerged as a key innate immune defense against intracellular pathogens. Autophagy mediates degradation of cytoplasmic contents within lysosomes and is highly conserved in eukaryotic cells (Levine and Deretic, 2007). This process can be subdivided into three types: chaperone-mediated autophagy (CMA), microautophagy, and macroautophagy (reviewed in Mizushima *et al.*, 2008). Macroautophagy, hereafter referred to as autophagy, is characterized by the presence of double-membrane vesicles termed autophagosomes, which bear the autophagy marker, microtubule-associated protein light chain 3 (LC3) (reviewed in Hussey *et al.*, 2009). Autophagy can target specific cargoes, including intracellular pathogens, resulting in their clearance in the lysosome (reviewed in Deretic and Levine, 2009; Hussey *et al.*, 2009). Autophagy has been shown to target bacterial pathogens within intact phagosomes, damaged phagosomes, and in the cytosol (Shahnazari and Brumell, 2011). Therefore, *L. monocytogenes* must successfully evade killing by the autophagy system at all stages of its residence within host cells. Below, we discuss the interactions of *L. monocytogenes* with the autophagy system and their outcome for infection by these bacteria.

2. PHAGOSOME ESCAPE

In order for *L. monocytogenes* to replicate in the cytosol, the bacterium must first escape from the phagosome. Numerous studies indicate that the initial phagosome escape requires both bacterial and host factors (Fig. 2.1). Escape to the cytosol can occur as rapidly as 30 min after bacterial entry (Beauregard *et al.*, 1997; Henry *et al.*, 2006). In murine macrophages, *L. monocytogenes* escape from $Rab7^{+}$, phosphatidylinositol 3-phosphate $(PI(3)P)^{+}$, $LAMP\text{-}1^{-}$ phagosomes (Henry *et al.*, 2006). Despite the fact that some bacterial factors have been identified that facilitate phagosome escape, the precise mechanism and the role of host factors is still undefined. It is likely that there is a dynamic interplay between bacterial factors perforating or altering the phagosomal membrane, and host factors being recruited to repair the phagosome which possibly inadvertently aid in bacterial escape.

2.1. Bacterial factors

The primary bacterial factor that mediates phagosome escape in macrophages is the cholesterol-dependent, pore-forming cytolysin LLO (Cossart *et al.*, 1989; Portnoy *et al.*, 1988, 1992a). Studies have shown that mutants lacking LLO cannot escape macrophage phagosomes (Birmingham *et al.*, 2008; Portnoy *et al.*, 1988). Within minutes of phagosome uptake, LLO can make pores in the phagosomal membrane (Beauregard *et al.*, 1997). These pores grow in size in a time-dependent manner which is evidenced by the exchange of fluorescent molecules of increasing sizes (Shaughnessy *et al.*, 2006). Therefore, LLO creates pores that gradually increase in size and become large enough to allow the exchange of proteins with the cytosol (Higgins *et al.*, 1999). Phagosome perforation also allows the exchange of protons and calcium ions with the cytosol, causing an increased pH and decreased Ca^{2+} concentration within the phagosomal compartment (Shaughnessy *et al.*, 2006). However, it has been shown that LLO requires an acidic pH for optimal activity

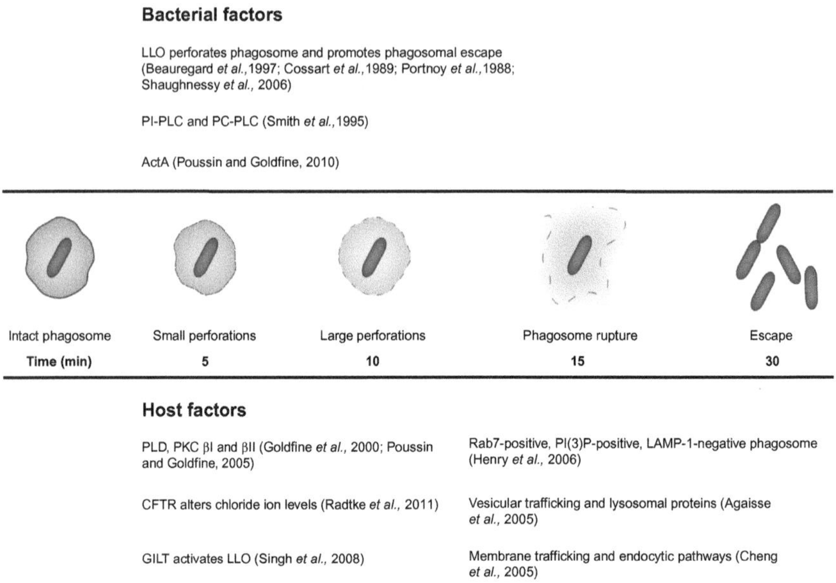

FIGURE 2.1 Kinetics of phagosome escape by *L. monocytogenes* during infection of macrophages. Perforations in the phagosome increase in size until the rupture of the phagosome, facilitating *L. monocytogenes* escape to the cytosol. Escape of *L. monocytogenes* from a macrophage phagosome is dependent on LLO, yet other bacterial and host factors can contribute to phagosome escape. (For color version of this figure, the reader is referred to the Web version of this chapter.)

(Glomski *et al.*, 2002; Portnoy *et al.*, 1992b) and that inhibition of acidification of the phagosome by treatment with bafilomycin A1 decreases *L. monocytogenes* escape from the phagosome (Beauregard *et al.*, 1997). Perhaps initial pore formation requires an acidic pH for LLO to permeabilize the membrane, after which the pH is neutralized by the exchange of ions through pores in the phagosomal membrane.

Two C-type phospholipases, phosphatidylinositol-specific (PI-PLC) and a broad-range phosphatidylcholine (PC-PLC), also help to mediate *L. monocytogenes* escape from the phagosome, possibly by digesting the phagosomal membrane. While LLO is necessary and sufficient for escape, the PLCs play a supporting role to allow for efficient bacterial escape (Shaughnessy *et al.*, 2006; Smith *et al.*, 1995). In addition to its direct role in permeabilizing the phagosomal membrane, PI-PLC can also mediate the translocation of host protein kinase C (PKC) βI and βII (Poussin and Goldfine, 2005). The consequence of PKC βI and βII downstream signaling can promote *L. monocytogenes* escape as inhibition of host PKCs can limit bacterial escape (Poussin *et al.*, 2009; Wadsworth and Goldfine, 1999, 2002). Therefore, LLO and PI-PLC activity, as well as host PKC pathways can act in concert to promote phagosome permeabilization and subsequent *L. monocytogenes* phagosome escape. It must be noted that the reverse is true for *L. monocytogenes* escape from the phagosome in human epithelial cells as the PLCs are sufficient for phagosome escape while LLO may be dispensable (Burrack *et al.*, 2009; Gründling *et al.*, 2003). It is currently unclear why different bacterial virulence factors are required for escape from the phagosome in different cell types. However, it is worth noting that LLO is sufficient to activate host phospholipases C and D during infection of macrophages (discussed below). Therefore, LLO may activate a host signaling pathway in macrophages that is sufficient to complement loss of bacterial PLCs in this cell type to promote phagosome escape.

Recently, the bacterial factor ActA has been implicated in phagosome escape (Poussin and Goldfine, 2010). The study of phagosome escape was enabled by a probe encoding the cell wall-binding domain of the Listeriophage endolysin Ply118 fused to yellow fluorescent protein (CBD-YFP; see Henry *et al.*, 2006). This probe allows detection of bacteria as soon as they have ruptured the phagosome sufficiently to allow access of the cytosolic probe to bacteria (Henry *et al.*, 2006). Using the CBD-YFP probe, ActA, a bacterial protein previously thought to be involved in actin-based motility and spreading exclusively in the cytosol, was shown to contribute to phagosome escape (Poussin and Goldfine, 2010). The observation that ActA has a role in phagosome escape leads to new hypotheses: *L. monocytogenes* could conceivably be within a phagosome and use ActA to recruit actin through large LLO and PLC derived pores, which could influence escape (Poussin and Goldfine, 2010). Alternatively, escape may be mediated by unknown protein–protein interactions of ActA (Poussin and Goldfine, 2010). It is worth noting that expression of ActA is thought to occur exclusively in the cytosol (Freitag and Jacobs, 1999). Therefore, the question of why Δ*actA* mutants are impaired in phagosome escape requires further study.

2.2. Host factors facilitating escape from the phagosome

In addition to its bacterial virulence factors, *L. monocytogenes* also requires host factors to assist in bacterial escape from the phagosome. PI-PLC can produce the signaling molecule diacylglycerol (DAG) and inositol phosphate upon cleavage of phosphatidylinositol (Griffith and Ryan, 1999). Despite using a *L. monocytogenes* strain lacking both bacterial PLCs, infection of macrophages resulted in an increased level of intracellular DAG over that of the uninfected cell. This observation indicated that *L. monocytogenes* could modulate DAG levels by activating host PLCs as well as utilizing bacterial PLCs (Smith *et al.*, 1995). Consistent with this idea, host phospholipase C (PLC) and phospholipase D (PLD) were found to be recruited to *L. monocytogenes* containing phagosomes in a manner that is dependent on LLO expression (Goldfine *et al.*, 2000). Further, treatment of cells with a PLD inhibitor reduced phagosome escape, suggesting a link between PLD activity and LLO-mediated escape from the phagosome (Goldfine *et al.*, 2000).

Another host factor, γ-interferon-inducible lysosomal thiol reductase (GILT) is necessary for activation of LLO leading to phagosome escape (Singh *et al.*, 2008). LLO requires activation by GILT via a thiol reductase mechanism in order to form pores and mediate *L. monocytogenes* phagosome escape (Singh *et al.*, 2008). GILT-deficient mice are protected from *L. monocytogenes* infection (Singh *et al.*, 2008). Given that LLO activity is tightly regulated (Schnupf, 2006, 2007), the requirement for a phagosomal protein, GILT, to activate LLO may be an additional bacterial fail-safe mechanism to limit LLO activity to that of the phagosome (Lam and Brumell, 2008).

The cystic fibrosis transmembrane conductance regulator (CFTR) is also reported to be required for phagosome escape by *L. monocytogenes* (Radtke *et al.*, 2011). CFTR is thought to increase the chloride ion concentration in the phagosome, and this may act in concert with LLO to facilitate escape possibly through changes in ion homeostasis (Radtke *et al.*, 2011). How chloride ions facilitate LLO activity in the phagosome remains unclear.

Finally, high-throughput RNA interference (RNAi) screens using macrophage-like *Drosophila* SL2 or S2 cells uncovered a number of additional host factors involved in mediating *L. monocytogenes* phagosome escape. In SL2 cells, host genes involved in vesicular trafficking and lysosomal transport were shown to aid in *L. monocytogenes* escape (Agaisse *et al.*, 2005). Cheng *et al.* (2005) performed an RNAi screen in S2 cells and looked for host genes that affected vacuolar escape in both an LLO-dependent and an LLO-independent manner. Host factors affecting phagosome escape in an LLO-dependent manner included those involved in membrane trafficking and endocytotic pathways (Cheng *et al.*, 2005). A second screen was performed to identify host targets of LLO that can be modulated to allow bacterial escape even in absence of LLO expression (Cheng *et al.*, 2005). When infected with an LLO-deficient mutant, knockdown of host genes involved in late stages of vesicular trafficking allowed vacuolar escape (Cheng *et al.*, 2005). Similar findings were reported in HEK293 cells (Burrack *et al.*, 2009). Therefore, these screens shed light on host factors that aid in *L. monocytogenes* phagosomal escape, both in the presence or absence of LLO expression.

3. AUTOPHAGY AND *L. MONOCYTOGENES*

The importance of autophagy in limiting *L. monocytogenes* replication has been demonstrated *in vivo*. Mice with Atg5-deficient macrophages ($Atg5^{flox/flox}$-Lyz-Cre) exhibit a 50% drop in survival 21 days p.i. with

L. monocytogenes when compared to wild-type mice (Zhao *et al.*, 2008). In particular, significantly greater bacterial load was observed in the livers at day 3 p.i. of the Atg5$^{flox/flox}$-Lyz-Cre mice when compared to control. Further, *Drosophila* mutants deficient in Atg5 or the pattern-recognition receptor, peptidoglycan recognition protein (PGRP)-LE, fail to induce autophagy in response to *L. monocytogenes* infection (Yano *et al.*, 2008). PGRP-LE recognition of the *L. monocytogenes* cell wall component, diaminopimelic acid-type peptidoglycan, results in autophagy targeting of *L. monocytogenes*, as assessed by increased LC3$^+$ double-membrane *L. monocytogenes* containing compartments (Yano *et al.*, 2008). *Drosophila* lacking in PGRP-LE or expressing a mutant PGRP-LE was unable to induce autophagy, resulting in increased susceptibility to *L. monocytogenes* infection. This results in a four-fold decrease in the number of surviving *Drosophila* mutants 8 d p.i. over the wild type (Yano *et al.*, 2008). Thus, these *in vivo* studies provide strong evidence that autophagic induction during *L. monocytogenes* infection is a critical host defense against the bacteria.

In vitro studies have revealed a complex picture of how LC3 targets *L. monocytogenes*. Depending on the stage of infection or where the bacteria are located in the host cell, LC3 targeting of *L. monocytogenes* may be mediated via different mechanisms. Approximately 35% of intracellular *L. monocytogenes* in RAW264.7 macrophages are targeted by LC3, with the peak of LC3 colocalizing with bacteria in the early stages of infection 1 h post infection (p.i.) (Birmingham *et al.*, 2007; Meyer-Morse *et al.*, 2010; Py *et al.*, 2007). LC3 targeting at 1 h p.i. in murine macrophages was found to be dependent on LLO as LLO-deficient *L. monocytogenes* does not become significantly LC3$^+$ at any point during infection (Birmingham *et al.*, 2007; Meyer-Morse *et al.*, 2010; Py *et al.*, 2007).

During later stages of infection of macrophages at 8 h p.i., when most bacteria are present in the cytosol, only 10% of wild type and ActA-deficient *L. monocytogenes* are LC3$^+$. Interestingly, while Δ*actA* mutants treated with the bacteriostatic agent, chloramphenicol, become 30% LC3$^+$, wild-type *L. monocytogenes* treated with chloramphenicol remain 10% LC3$^+$ (Birmingham *et al.*, 2007). This data suggests that cytosolic autophagy targeting of *L. monocytogenes* may be evaded by expression of ActA (Birmingham *et al.*, 2007; Rich *et al.*, 2003). It must be noted that LC3 targeting of Δ*actA* mutants have been reported to occur even in absence of chloramphenicol treatment (Yoshikawa *et al.*, 2009). This difference may be explained by the fact that different genetic backgrounds were used in these studies. Thus, it appears that different strains of wild-type *L. monocytogenes* may have different kinetics of LC3 targeting.

Despite the complexity of different bacterial backgrounds, it is clear that ActA plays a role in *L. monocytogenes* avoidance of autophagy targeting. It is known that the Δ*actA* mutant colocalizes with ubiquitinated proteins (Ub) at 8 h p.i. (Perrin *et al.*, 2004). Recent work by Sasakawa and colleagues suggests that this protein ubiquitination event mediates recruitment of adaptor proteins such as p62/SQSTM1, which leads to autophagic targeting of the Δ*actA* mutant (Yoshikawa *et al.*, 2009). Another adaptor, NDP52, has also been implicated in the autophagy targeting of cytosolic *L. monocytogenes* (Mostowy *et al.*, 2011). Thus, these combined observations suggest that ActA may play a critical role in evading autophagy targeting by preventing ubiquitination of *L. monocytogenes* in the cytosol. Further, recent findings suggest that in conjunction with ActA, another bacterial effector, InlK, is also involved in the avoidance of autophagy targeting in the cytosol (Dortet *et al.*, 2011). InlK is thought to mediate recruitment of major vault protein to the bacterial surface, serving as a molecular "shield" to prevent targeting by autophagy.

L. monocytogenes mutants deficient in PI-PLC exhibit markedly greater bacterial replication in Atg5-deficient MEFs when compared to wild-type MEFs (Birmingham *et al.*, 2007). This observation suggests that PI-PLC, or perhaps both bacterial PLCs, may also play a role in the evasion of autophagy that is currently unappreciated. Thus, there may be multiple mechanisms employed by *L. monocytogenes* to evade LC3 targeting within host cells.

Current data suggests a possible scenario whereby *L. monocytogenes* is subject to two independent LC3-targeting events at different stages of infection. At 1 h p.i. of murine macrophages, where the majority of *L. monocytogenes* are still inside phagosomes, one-third of the population is targeted by LC3 (Fig. 2.2A). It is unclear how this targeting occurs and if protein ubiquitination plays a role in early LC3 targeting. Early LC3 targeting of *L. monocytogenes* may result in bacterial clearance. Data indicates that it can also lead to the formation of SLAPs (*S*pacious *L*isteria-containing *P*hagosomes). SLAPs are large, non-degradative LAMP-1$^+$, and LC3$^+$ vacuoles that contain *L. monocytogenes* (Birmingham *et al.*, 2008). Since the formation of SLAPs was found to require autophagy in the host cell and expression of LLO by bacteria, it has been proposed that SLAPs represent a "stalemate" between the host and bacteria, allowing slow bacterial replication in SLAPs that may allow chronic *L. monocytogenes* infection in a host (Birmingham *et al.*, 2008). Indeed, compartments resembling SLAPs have been observed in a severe combined immunodeficiency (SCID) mouse model of *L. monocytogenes* chronic infection (Bhardwaj *et al.*, 1998). Thus, early LC3 targeting of *L. monocytogenes* results either in bacterial clearance or in SLAP formation which may promote chronic infection. After entry into the cytosol, wild-type bacteria utilize ActA to inhibit their ubiquitination by host E3 ligases and thereby are not targeted by autophagy (Fig. 2.2B). ActA also mediates actin-based motility and spread to neighboring cells. Expression of ActA on the

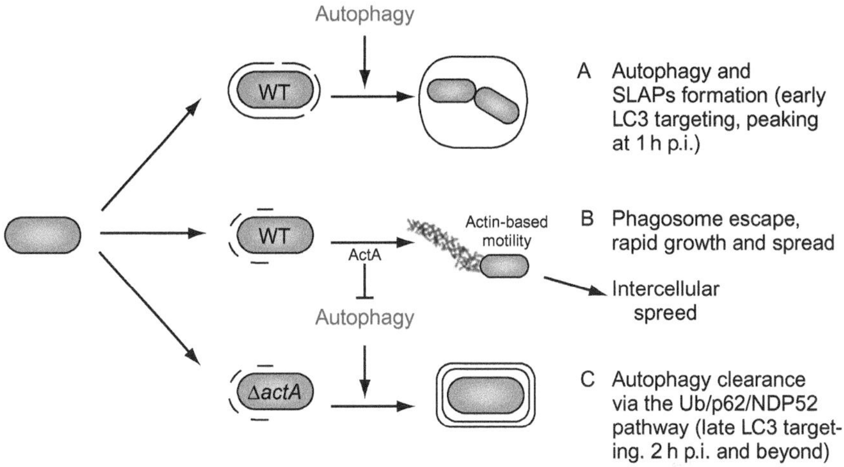

FIGURE 2.2 Pathways of autophagy targeting of intracellular *L. monocytogenes* in murine macrophages. (A) Early LC3 targeting of *L. monocytogenes* which peaks at 1 h p.i. (B) As the infection progresses, wild-type *L. monocytogenes* escapes from the phagosome and, via the activity of ActA, prevents ubiquitination, thus avoiding autophagy targeting in the cytosol. (C) *L. monocytogenes* lacking ActA expression cannot prevent ubiquitination. As such, Δ*actA L. monocytogenes* is ubiquitinated and targeted for autophagy clearance.

bacterial surface may involve a significant delay after escape from the phagosome (Freitag and Jacobs, 1999). During this window of time, bacteria may employ other factors such as InlK and PLCs to evade autophagy. It is also possible that a subset of these bacteria do not express ActA fast enough to prevent bacterial ubiquitination, leading to recruitment of adaptor proteins such as p62 or NDP52, and targeting of bacteria to autophagy (Fig. 2.2C).

4. CONCLUSION

The fate of *L. monocytogenes* inside a macrophage depends on both bacterial factors (LLO, PLCs, and ActA) and host factors (autophagy), giving rise to different populations of *L. monocytogenes* that experience different intracellular fates (Fig. 2.2). While one population of *L. monocytogenes* escape from the phagosome and participate in acute bacterial infection, replication, and cell-to-cell spread, another population of *L. monocytogenes* that is targeted by LC3 gives rise to SLAPs which may be important for chronic infections. The evolution of bacterial strategies for both acute and chronic infection may not be limited to *L. monocytogenes*. SLAP-like structures have also been observed for other intracellular bacteria including

Staphylococcus aureus (Kubica *et al.*, 2008), *Yersinia pestis* (Pujol *et al.*, 2009), *Helicobacter pylori* (Allen *et al.*, 2005), as well as Uropathogenic *Escherichia coli* (UPEC) (Kerrn *et al.*, 2005; Mysorekar and Hultgren, 2006). Thus, the use of *L. monocytogenes* as a model intracellular pathogen may provide insight into how other bacterial pathogens escape from the phagosome or persist in vacuoles inside host cells.

REFERENCES

Agaisse, H., Burrack, L. S., Philips, J. A., Rubin, E. J., Perrimon, N., and Higgins, D. E. (2005). Genome-wide RNAi screen for host factors required for intracellular bacterial infection. *Science* **309,** 1248–1251.

Allen, L. A., Beecher, B. R., Lynch, J. T., Rohner, O. V., and Wittine, L. M. (2005). Helicobacter pylori disrupts NADPH oxidase targeting in human neutrophils to induce extracellular superoxide release. *J. Immunol.* **174,** 3658–3667.

Beauregard, K. E., Lee, K. D., Collier, R. J., and Swanson, J. A. (1997). pH-dependent perforation of macrophage phagosomes by listeriolysin O from Listeria monocytogenes. *J. Exp. Med.* **186,** 1159–1163.

Bhardwaj, V., Kanagawa, O., Swanson, P. E., and Unanue, E. R. (1998). Chronic Listeria infection in SCID mice: Requirements for the carrier state and the dual role of T cells in transferring protection or suppression. *J. Immunol.* **160,** 376–384.

Birmingham, C. L., Canadien, V., Gouin, E., Troy, E. B., Yoshimori, T., Cossart, P., Higgins, D. E., and Brumell, J. H. (2007). Listeria monocytogenes evades killing by autophagy during colonization of host cells. *Autophagy* **3,** 442–451.

Birmingham, C. L., Canadien, V., Kaniuk, N. A., Steinberg, B. E., Higgins, D. E., and Brumell, J. H. (2008). Listeriolysin O allows *Listeria monocytogenes* replication in macrophage vacuoles. *Nature* **451,** 350–354.

Burrack, L. S., Harper, J. W., and Higgins, D. E. (2009). Perturbation of vacuolar maturation promotes listeriolysin O-independent vacuolar escape during Listeria monocytogenes infection of human cells. *Cell. Microbiol.* **11,** 1382–1398.

Cheng, L. W., Viala, J. P., Stuurman, N., Wiedemann, U., Vale, R. D., and Portnoy, D. A. (2005). Use of RNA interference in *Drosophila* S2 cells to identify host pathways controlling compartmentalization of an intracellular pathogen. *Proc. Natl. Acad. Sci. USA* **102,** 13646–13651.

Cossart, P., Vicente, M. F., Mengaud, J., Baquero, F., Perez-Diaz, J. C., and Berche, P. (1989). Listeriolysin O is essential for virulence of *Listeria monocytogenes*: Direct evidence obtained by gene complementation. *Infect. Immun.* **57,** 3629–3636.

Deretic, V., and Levine, B. (2009). Autophagy, immunity, and microbial adaptations. *Cell Host Microbe* **5,** 527–549.

Dortet, L., Mostowy, S., Louaka, A. S., Gouin, E., Nahori, M. A., Wiemer, E. A., Dussurget, O., and Cossart, P. (2011). Recruitment of the major vault protein by InlK: A Listeria monocytogenes strategy to avoid autophagy. *PLoS Pathog.* **7,** e1002168.

Flannagan, R. S., Cosio, G., and Grinstein, S. (2009). Antimicrobial mechanisms of phagocytes and bacterial evasion strategies. *Nat. Rev. Microbiol.* **7,** 355–366.

Freitag, N. E., and Jacobs, K. E. (1999). Examination of Listeria monocytogenes intracellular gene expression by using the green fluorescent protein of Aequorea victoria. *Infect. Immun.* **67,** 1844–1852.

Glomski, I. J., Gedde, M. M., Tsang, A. W., Swanson, J. A., and Portnoy, D. A. (2002). The *Listeria monocytogenes* hemolysin has an acidic pH optimum to compartmentalize activity and prevent damage to infected host cells. *J. Cell Biol.* **156,** 1029–1038.

Goldfine, H., Wadsworth, S. J., and Johnston, N. C. (2000). Activation of host phospholipases C and D in macrophages after infection with *Listeria monocytogenes*. *Infect. Immun.* **68,** 5735–5741.

Griffith, O. H., and Ryan, M. (1999). Bacterial phosphatidylinositol-specific phospholipase C: Structure, function, and interaction with lipids. *Biochim. Biophys. Acta* **1441,** 237–254.

Gründling, A., Gonzalez, M. D., and Higgins, D. E. (2003). Requirement of the *Listeria monocytogenes* broad-range phospholipase PC-PLC during infection of human epithelial cells. *J. Bacteriol.* **185,** 6295–6307.

Henry, R., Shaughnessy, L., Loessner, M. J., Alberti-Segui, C., Higgins, D. E., and Swanson, J. A. (2006). Cytolysin-dependent delay of phagosome maturation in macrophages infected with Listeria monocytogenes. *Cell. Microbiol.* **8,** 107–119.

Higgins, D. E., Shastri, N., and Portnoy, D. A. (1999). Delivery of protein to the cytosol of macrophages using *Escherichia coli* K-12. *Mol. Microbiol.* **31,** 1631–1641.

Hussey, S., Travassos, L. H., and Jones, N. L. (2009). Autophagy as an emerging dimension to adaptive and innate immunity. *Semin. Immunol.* **21,** 233–241.

Kerrn, M. B., Struve, C., Blom, J., Frimodt-Moller, N., and Krogfelt, K. A. (2005). Intracellular persistence of Escherichia coli in urinary bladders from mecillinam-treated mice. *J. Antimicrob. Chemother.* **55,** 383–386.

Kirkegaard, K., Taylor, M. P., and Jackson, W. T. (2004). Cellular autophagy: Surrender, avoidance and subversion by microorganisms. *Nat. Rev. Microbiol.* **2,** 301–314.

Kubica, M., Guzik, K., Koziel, J., Zarebski, M., Richter, W., Gajkowska, B., Golda, A., Maciag-Gudowska, A., Brix, K., Shaw, L., *et al.* (2008). A potential new pathway for Staphylococcus aureus dissemination: The silent survival of *S. aureus* phagocytosed by human monocyte-derived macrophages. *PLoS One* **3,** e1409.

Kumar, Y., and Valdivia, R. H. (2009). Leading a sheltered life: Intracellular pathogens and maintenance of vacuolar compartments. *Cell Host Microbe* **5,** 593–601.

Lam, G. Y., and Brumell, J. H. (2008). Cell biology: A Listeria escape trick. *Nature* **455,** 1186–1187.

Levine, B., and Deretic, V. (2007). Unveiling the roles of autophagy in innate and adaptive immunity. *Nat. Rev. Immunol.* **7,** 767–777.

Meyer-Morse, N., Robbins, J. R., Rae, C. S., Mochegova, S. N., Swanson, M. S., Zhao, Z., Virgin, H. W., and Portnoy, D. (2010). Listeriolysin O is necessary and sufficient to induce autophagy during Listeria monocytogenes infection. *PLoS One* **5,** e8610.

Mizushima, N., Levine, B., Cuervo, A. M., and Klionsky, D. J. (2008). Autophagy fights disease through cellular self-digestion. *Nature* **451,** 1069–1075.

Mostowy, S., Sancho-Shimizu, V., Hamon, M. A., Simeone, R., Brosch, R., Johansen, T., and Cossart, P. (2011). p62 and NDP52 proteins target intracytosolic Shigella and Listeria to different autophagy pathways. *J. Biol. Chem.* **286,** 26987–26995.

Mysorekar, I. U., and Hultgren, S. J. (2006). Mechanisms of uropathogenic Escherichia coli persistence and eradication from the urinary tract. *Proc. Natl. Acad. Sci. USA* **103,** 14170–14175.

Perrin, A. J., Jiang, X., Birmingham, C. L., So, N. S., and Brumell, J. H. (2004). Recognition of bacteria in the cytosol of Mammalian cells by the ubiquitin system. *Curr. Biol.* **14,** 806–811.

Portnoy, D. A., Jacks, P. S., and Hinrichs, D. J. (1988). Role of hemolysin for the intracellular growth of *Listeria monocytogenes*. *J. Exp. Med.* **167,** 1459–1471.

Portnoy, D. A., Chakraborty, T., Goebel, W., and Cossart, P. (1992a). Molecular determinants of *Listeria monocytogenes* pathogenesis. *Infect. Immun.* **60,** 1263–1267.

Portnoy, D. A., Tweten, R. K., Kehoe, M., and Bielecki, J. (1992b). Capacity of listeriolysin O, streptolysin O, and perfringolysin O to mediate growth of *Bacillus subtilis* within mammalian cells. *Infect. Immun.* **60,** 2710–2717.

Poussin, M. A., and Goldfine, H. (2005). Involvement of *Listeria monocytogenes* phosphatidylinositol-specific phospholipase C and host protein kinase C in permeabilization of the macrophage phagosome. *Infect. Immun.* **73,** 4410–4413.

Poussin, M. A., and Goldfine, H. (2010). Evidence for the involvement of ActA in maturation of the *Listeria monocytogenes* phagosome. *Cell Res.* **20,** 109–112.

Poussin, M. A., Leitges, M., and Goldfine, H. (2009). The ability of *Listeria monocytogenes* PI-PLC to facilitate escape from the macrophage phagosome is dependent on host PKCbeta. *Microb. Pathog.* **46,** 1–5.

Pujol, C., Klein, K. A., Romanov, G. A., Palmer, L. E., Cirota, C., Zhao, Z., and Bliska, J. B. (2009). Yersinia pestis can reside in autophagosomes and avoid xenophagy in murine macrophages by preventing vacuole acidification. *Infect. Immun.* **77,** 2251–2261.

Py, B. F., Lipinski, M. M., and Yuan, J. (2007). Autophagy limits Listeria monocytogenes intracellular growth in the early phase of primary infection. *Autophagy* **3,** 117–125.

Radtke, A. L., Anderson, K. L., Davis, M. J., DiMagno, M. J., Swanson, J. A., and O'Riordan, M. X. (2011). *Listeria monocytogenes* exploits cystic fibrosis transmembrane conductance regulator (CFTR) to escape the phagosome. *Proc. Natl. Acad. Sci. USA* **108,** 1633–1638.

Rich, K. A., Burkett, C., and Webster, P. (2003). Cytoplasmic bacteria can be targets for autophagy. *Cell. Microbiol.* **5,** 455–468.

Rocourt, J., and Bille, J. (1997). Foodborne listeriosis. *World Health Stat. Q.* **50,** 67–73.

Schnupf, P., Portnoy, D. A., and Decatur, A. L. (2006). Phosphorylation, ubiquitination and degradation of listeriolysin O in mammalian cells: Role of the PEST-like sequence. *Cell. Microbiol.* **8,** 353–364.

Schnupf, P., Zhou, J., Varshavsky, A., and Portnoy, D. A. (2007). Listeriolysin O secreted by Listeria monocytogenes into the host cell cytosol is degraded by the N-end rule pathway. *Infect. Immun.* **75,** 5135–5147.

Shahnazari, S., and Brumell, J. H. (2011). Mechanisms and consequences of bacterial targeting by the autophagy pathway. *Curr. Opin. Microbiol.* **14,** 68–75.

Shaughnessy, L. M., Hoppe, A. D., Christensen, K. A., and Swanson, J. A. (2006). Membrane perforations inhibit lysosome fusion by altering pH and calcium in Listeria monocytogenes phagosomes. *Cell. Microbiol.* **8,** 781–792.

Singh, R., Jamieson, A., and Cresswell, P. (2008). GILT is a critical host factor for *Listeria monocytogenes infection*. *Nature* **455,** 1244–1247.

Smith, G. A., Marquis, H., Jones, S., Johnston, N. C., Portnoy, D. A., and Goldfine, H. (1995). The two distinct phospholipases C of *Listeria monocytogenes* have overlapping roles in escape from a vacuole and cell-to-cell spread. *Infect. Immun.* **63,** 4231–4237.

Tilney, L. G., and Portnoy, D. A. (1989). Actin filaments and the growth, movement, and spread of the intracellular bacterial parasite, Listeria monocytogenes. *J. Cell Biol.* **109,** 597–1608.

Wadsworth, S. J., and Goldfine, H. (1999). *Listeria monocytogenes* phospholipase C-dependent calcium signaling modulates bacterial entry into J774 macrophage-like cells. *Infect. Immun.* **67,** 1770–1778.

Wadsworth, S. J., and Goldfine, H. (2002). Mobilization of protein kinase C in macrophages induced by Listeria monocytogenes affects its internalization and escape from the phagosome. *Infect. Immun.* **70,** 4650–4660.

Yano, T., Mita, S., Ohmori, H., Oshima, Y., Fujimoto, Y., Ueda, R., Takada, H., Goldman, W. E., Fukase, K., Silverman, N., *et al.* (2008). Autophagic control of Listeria through intracellular innate immune recognition in drosophila. *Nat. Immunol.* **9,** 908–916.

Yoshikawa, Y., Ogawa, M., Hain, T., Yoshida, M., Fukumatsu, M., Kim, M., Mimuro, H., Nakagawa, I., Yanagawa, T., Ishii, T., *et al.* (2009). Listeria monocytogenes ActA-mediated escape from autophagic recognition. *Nat. Cell Biol.* **11,** 1233–1240.

Zhao, Z., Fux, B., Goodwin, M., Dunay, I. R., Strong, D., Miller, B. C., Cadwell, K., Delgado, M. A., Ponpuak, M., Green, K. G., *et al.* (2008). Autophagosome-independent essential function for the autophagy protein Atg5 in cellular immunity to intracellular pathogens. *Cell Host Microbe* **4,** 458–469.

CHAPTER 3

Virulence Factors That Modulate the Cell Biology of *Listeria* Infection and the Host Response

Serge Mostowy[*,†,‡] and **Pascale Cossart**[*,†,‡]

Contents

Abstract

The Gram-positive bacterial pathogen *Listeria monocytogenes* has become one of the best studied models in infection biology. This review will update our knowledge of *Listeria* virulence factors and highlight their role during the *Listeria* infection process.

* Institut Pasteur, Unité des Interactions Bactéries-Cellules, Paris, France
† Inserm, U604, Paris, France
‡ INRA, USC2020, Paris, France

Advances in Immunology, Volume 113
ISSN 0065-2776, DOI: 10.1016/B978-0-12-394590-7.00007-5

1. INTRODUCTION

The molecular basis of *Listeria* pathogenesis has been analyzed for more than two decades. Cell biology approaches have revealed the strategies used by *Listeria* to enter into nonphagocytic cells, to escape from the internalization vacuole, to circumvent host immune responses and move intracellularly, and to spread from cell to cell (Fig. 3.1). These studies have been instrumental to understand the infection process *in vivo*.

In this review, we update our knowledge of *Listeria* virulence factors (Table 3.1) and discuss a selection of recent cell biological insights gained from studying *Listeria* pathogenesis. We first focus on the "mechanics" of the infection, that is, rearrangements of the cytoskeleton during entry into cells or cell-to-cell spread, and then highlight emerging aspects of the host response to infection that *Listeria* is directly able to manipulate, that is, autophagy, posttranslational modifications, and epigenetic regulation of gene expression.

2. THE CELL BIOLOGY OF *LISTERIA* INFECTION

2.1. *Listeria* invasion and the new role for clathrin and septins

Listeria monocytogenes employs a variety of proteins, and in particular, members of a protein family known as the internalins, to adhere to and invade host cells. Internalins are members of the leucine rich repeat (LRR) superfamily, a diverse group of proteins characterized by tandem arrays of LRRs (Bierne and Cossart, 2007). The two major invasion proteins are internalin (InlA) and InlB. The receptor for InlA is E-cadherin (Mengaud *et al.*, 1996), and the receptors for InlB are gC1qR/p32 (the receptor for the globular part of complement component C1q), Met/hepatocyte growth factor (HGF) receptor, and glycosaminoglycans (Braun *et al.*, 2000; Jonquières *et al.*, 2001; Shen *et al.*, 2000).

The mechanisms underlying the actin rearrangements required for *Listeria* invasion into nonphagocytic cells have been examined in depth (Bierne and Cossart, 2002; Cossart *et al.*, 2003; Pizarro-Cerda and Cossart, 2006, 2009). An important finding has been the recent discovery that clathrin, a molecule thought to be only involved in internalization of macromolecules, was involved in the entry of *Listeria* (Veiga and Cossart, 2005; Veiga *et al.*, 2007). Clathrin-coated vesicles arise from the self-polymerization of clathrin into a lattice around budding vesicles (Sorkin, 2004). Clathrin in coated vesicles is structured as a triskelion with three heavy (192 kDa) and three light (25–29 kDa) chains that bind to each other in a polyhedral lattice (Fotin *et al.*, 2004). At the site of *Listeria*

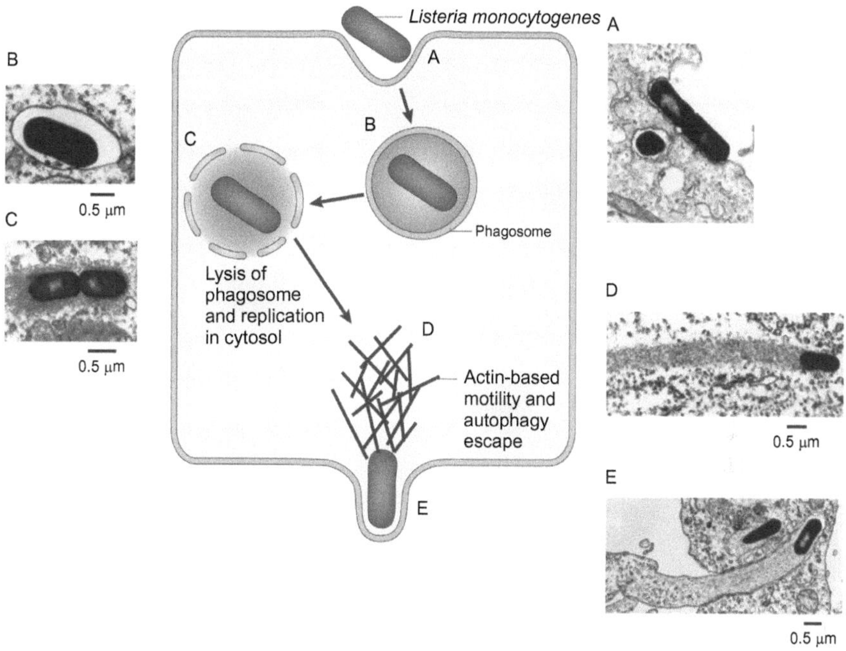

FIGURE 3.1 The intracellular lifestyle of *Listeria monocytogenes*. Schematic representation and electron micrographs of the *L. monocytogenes* life cycle. (A) *L. monocytogenes* induces its entry into a nonprofessional phagocyte. (B) Bacteria are internalized in a phagosome. (C and D) The membrane of the phagocytic vacuole is disrupted by the secretion of LLO and phospholipases. Bacteria are released into the cytosol where they start to polymerize actin and avoid autophagy, as observed by the presence of actin tails. (E) Actin polymerization allows bacteria to propel into a neighboring cell by forming protrusions in the plasma membrane. This figure is reproduced with permission from Hamon *et al.* (2006). (See Color Insert.)

entry, clathrin is recruited and its assembly requires the ubiquitin ligase Cbl (which ubiquitinates Met) or Hakai (which ubiquitinates E-cadherin). The involvement of clathrin in bacterial entry has challenged the prevailing dogma that particles exceeding 150 nm cannot be internalized through a clathrin-dependent mechanism (Conner and Schmid, 2003). RNA interference experiments have shown that clathrin assembly precedes actin rearrangements at the site of entry (Veiga and Cossart, 2005; Veiga *et al.*, 2007) where clathrin may act as a platform for the recruitment of proteins involved in the actin rearrangements required for entry (e.g., the adaptor proteins Dab2, Hip1R, and myosin VI; Bonazzi *et al.*, 2011). Interestingly, work done in non-infected cells has shown that actin dynamics counteract membrane tension during clathrin-mediated endocytosis (Boulant *et al.*, 2011), highlighting the

TABLE 3.1 Table of virulence factors that modulate the cell biology of *Listeria* infection and the host response

Gene name	Role	Reference
actA	Actin-based motility, autophagy evasion	Kocks *et al.* (1993), Welch *et al.* (1997), Yoshikawa *et al.* (2009)
hly (LLO)	Phagosome escape, transcriptional reprogramming, deSUMOylation, mitochondrial fragmentation	Shaughnessy *et al.* (2006), Hamon and Cossart (2007), Ribet *et al.* (2010), Stavru *et al.* (2011a)
inlA	Bacterial entry	Mengaud *et al.* (1996)
inlB	Bacterial entry, signaling molecule	Shen *et al.* (2000)
inlC	Protrusion formation, dampens innate immune response	Rajabian *et al.* (2009), Gouin *et al.* (2010)
inlK	Autophagy evasion	Dortet *et al.* (2011)
lntA	Chromatin remodeling	Lebreton *et al.* (2011)
oatA	Pepditoglycan modification	Aubry *et al.* (2011), Rae *et al.* (2011)
pgdA	Pepditoglycan modification	Boneca *et al.* (2007)
plcA (PI-PLC)	Vacuole escape	Smith *et al.* (1995)
plcB (PC-PLC)	Vacuole escape	Smith *et al.* (1995), Vazquez-Boland *et al.* (1992)

interdependent relationship between actin rearrangements and clathrin-mediated endocytosis. In support of this, the ultrastructural details of actin at sites of clathrin-mediated entry have recently been achieved (Collins *et al.*, 2011). However, the precise molecular connection between clathrin-mediated endocytosis and actin rearrangements during *Listeria* entry remains to be fully determined.

Septins have also been shown to play a critical role in bacterial entry. Septins are GTP-binding proteins of 30–65 kDa required in many organisms for the completion of cell division (Kinoshita, 2003; Weirich *et al.*, 2008). Septins associate with cellular membranes, actin filaments, and microtubules and are increasingly regarded as novel cytoskeletal components. Unlike actin and microtubules, septins assemble into nonpolar filaments (John *et al.*, 2007; Sirajuddin *et al.*, 2007) that orchestrate a variety of key cellular processes by serving as scaffolds for protein recruitment and/or diffusion barriers to compartmentalize discrete cellular domains (Saarikangas and Barral, 2011; Spiliotis and Gladfelter, 2011).

Although implicated in several human diseases (Hall and Russell, 2004), the molecular functions of septins are poorly understood because of the multiple septin genes (SEPT1 through SEPT14 in humans, but SEPT13 is a pseudogene) and their extensive splicing, and their different distribution in different cell types. In addition, septins form heteropolymers with the biologically active unit of human septins being a hetero-hexamer (Sirajuddin *et al.*, 2007) and/or a hetero-octamer (Sandrock *et al.*, 2011; Sellin *et al.*, 2011). In contrast to the well-established role of actin during *Listeria* invasion, septin function had not been addressed. It was recently shown that septins are recruited at the site of *Listeria* entry and strikingly form ring-like structures around the bacteria (Mostowy *et al.*, 2009b). RNA interference studies established that SEPT2, a septin required for filament formation (Sellin *et al.*, 2011; Sirajuddin *et al.*, 2007), significantly contributes to the bacterial entry process (Mostowy *et al.*, 2011a, 2009b). In contrast, SEPT11, a septin considered replaceable in certain cell types, appeared to restrict the process of internalization, highlighting different roles for different septins (Mostowy *et al.*, 2009a, 2011a). The accumulation of septins is intimately linked to the accumulation of $PI(4,5)P_2$ and actin at sites of phagocytosis, albeit in an unknown fashion (Huang *et al.*, 2008; Mostowy *et al.*, 2009b). The mechanisms underlying septin recruitment at the site of bacterial entry, and more generally how septin ring-like assembly is orchestrated with actin polymerization and clathrin coat formation requires further investigation.

2.2. Escape from the vacuole

Listeria survives intracellularly by modifying and escaping from phagosomes using a combination of effectors (Hamon *et al.*, 2006). This step is mainly mediated by the pore-forming and cholesterol-dependent toxin listeriolysin O (LLO) (Schnupf and Portnoy, 2007). LLO inhibits the maturation of phagosomes by creating pores in the phagosomal membrane which inhibit lysosome fusion by altering pH and calcium (Shaughnessy *et al.*, 2006). The contribution of host factors to *Listeria* phagosomal escape is incompletely defined. LLO needs to be activated by acidification and/or by the host enzyme GILT (IFNγ-inducible lysosomal thiol reductase) that is found inside the phagosome (Singh *et al.*, 2008). A recent report has shown that CFTR (cystic fibrosis transmembrane conductance regulator) increases chloride concentration inside the phagosome and potentiates LLO-mediated pore formation (Radtke *et al.*, 2011). In addition to LLO, *Listeria* expresses two membrane-active phospholipase C enzymes (i.e., PI-PLC and PC-PLC) that contribute to rupture the *Listeria*-containing phagosome and help bacteria escape to the cytosol (Smith *et al.*, 1995; Vazquez-Boland *et al.*, 1992).

Although thought to reside primarily in the cytosol, *L. monocytogenes* can replicate under some circumstances inside macrophage vacuoles called SLAPs (spacious *Listeria*-containing phagosomes) (Birmingham *et al.*, 2008). The formation of SLAPs only occurs upon impaired LLO production. The rate of bacterial replication inside SLAPs is reduced compared with bacterial replication in the cytosol, yet it could contribute to the development of chronic *Listeria* infection.

2.3. Actin-based motility and cell-to-cell spread

After escaping from the phagosome to the cytosol, *Listeria* has the ability to initiate actin-based motility (Gouin *et al.*, 2005). Actin polymerization propels the bacteria through the cytosol and into neighboring cells. Direct spread from cell to cell allows *Listeria* to circumvent host immune responses. The *L. monocytogenes* surface protein ActA mimics the host cell WASP family proteins, recruits the Arp2/3 complex (Welch *et al.*, 1997), and promotes actin polymerization to form actin tails (Kocks *et al.*, 1993). ActA is necessary for bacterial motility in tissue culture cells (Robbins *et al.*, 1999) and is critical for pathogenesis in the murine model of infection (Brundage *et al.*, 1993). ActA is sufficient for motility in the absence of other bacterial factors, as demonstrated by the observation that ActA-coated latex beads polymerize actin and undergo actin-based motility in cell extracts (Cameron *et al.*, 1999).

Despite the relatively few components required for actin-based motility of *Listeria in vitro* (Loisel *et al.*, 1999), a larger number of proteins are probably involved during the actin-based motility of *Listeria in vivo* (Van Troys *et al.*, 2008). Intriguingly, septins do not seem to significantly affect the speed of movement but do form rings around actin tails and the moving bacteria (Mostowy *et al.*, 2010). Interaction between InlC, a member of the *Listeria* internalin family highly expressed inside infected cells (Gouin *et al.*, 2010), and the actin-binding protein Tuba has been shown to promote protrusion formation and cell-to-cell spread (Rajabian *et al.*, 2009). Clearly, a complete picture of proteins and mechanisms regulating actin dynamics and movement *in vivo* has not been obtained. This will be critical for the complete understanding of infectious processes.

3. BACTERIAL INTERACTION WITH HOST DEFENSES

3.1. Escape from intracellular immunity

In the phagocytic vacuole or in the cytosol, *Listeria* can interact with a variety of host cell defense mechanisms (reviewed in Stavru *et al.*, 2011a). Recent work has highlighted the role of *Listeria* peptidoglycan modifying enzymes to evade innate immune responses. PgdA is an enzyme which deacetylates the *N*-acetylglucosamine residues of *L. monocytogenes* peptidoglycan and confers resistance to lysozyme (Boneca *et al.*, 2007).

PgdA mutants are rapidly destroyed in macrophage vacuoles and are among the most attenuated mutants of *L. monocytogenes*. OatA induces another peptidoglycan modification critical for the survival of *Listeria* in infected hosts (Aubry *et al.*, 2011; Rae *et al.*, 2011). Modification by OatA leads to the acetylation of muramic acid residues. Strikingly, the host cytokine response for the PgdA and the OatA mutants is different, indicating nonredundant roles for these two modifications (Aubry *et al.*, 2011).

3.2. Escape from autophagy

Autophagy is a process by which cytoplasmic materials are targeted to lysosomes for degradation (Levine and Kroemer, 2008; Mizushima *et al.*, 2008; Rubinsztein, 2006). Over 30 autophagy-related (Atg) genes have been identified in yeast, and mammalian homologues have been isolated and functionally characterized (He and Klionsky, 2009; Levine and Klionsky, 2004). Basal levels of autophagy ensure the maintenance of intracellular homeostasis, and many studies have revealed its key role in diverse cellular processes such as cellular stress, differentiation, development, and longevity (Levine and Klionsky, 2004; Vellai *et al.*, 2009). Autophagy is also linked to a wide range of disease states (Levine and Kroemer, 2008; Mizushima *et al.*, 2008; Shintani and Klionsky, 2004). Recent evidence has implicated the autophagic pathway in pathogenesis (Levine and Deretic, 2007; Levine *et al.*, 2011), and ubiquitination has emerged as central for autophagic recognition of intracytosolic pathogens (Mostowy *et al.*, 2011b; Thurston *et al.*, 2009; Wild *et al.*, 2011; Yoshikawa *et al.*, 2009). Ubiquitin-associated bacteria recognized by the autophagy machinery are trapped by autophagosomal membrane for delivery to lysosomes where they undergo degradation. The autophagy receptors p62 (SQSTM1) (Pankiv *et al.*, 2007), NDP52 (nuclear dot protein 52 kDa) (Thurston *et al.*, 2009), and OPTN (Wild *et al.*, 2011) are adaptor proteins directly involved in detecting ubiquitinated bacteria and targeting them to autophagy.

Several reports have shown a link between *Listeria* infection and autophagy. It was first noticed that unless *L. monocytogenes* were forming actin tails, autophagic markers could accumulate around intracytosolic bacteria (Birmingham *et al.*, 2007; Kathryn *et al.*, 2003; Perrin *et al.*, 2004). The underlying mechanism has recently been described. Independent of its ability to mediate bacterial motility, ActA recruits host proteins and disguises *Listeria* from ubiquitination and autophagic recognition (Mostowy *et al.*, 2011b; Yoshikawa *et al.*, 2009). Therefore, ActA mutants are targeted to autophagy, while ActA-expressing bacteria are not. InlK is another surface protein that contributes to listerial escape from autophagy (Dortet *et al.*, 2011). Instead of recruiting the actin polymerization machinery, *Listeria* expressing InlK recruits the major vault protein (MVP) to evade ubiquitination and autophagic recognition. *Listeria* could also co-opt autophagy processes. A wealth of evidence has implicated mitochondrial dynamics in pathogenesis (Rudel *et al.*, 2010; West *et al.*, 2011), and the autophagic turnover of mitochondria (mitophagy; reviewed in Green *et al.*, 2011) in response to mitochondrial fragmentation by LLO (Stavru *et al.*, 2011b) may be another critical feature of the host response to *Listeria* infection. The precise and probably multiple roles of autophagy in *Listeria* pathogenesis *in vivo* remain to be established.

3.3. Posttranslational modifications in infected cells

Posttranslational modifications are among the first events used by eukaryotic cells to react to infection (Ribet and Cossart, 2010). They provide a versatile mechanism for regulating a broad range of cellular processes, and posttranslational modifications of key proteins are increasingly recognized as important checkpoints during infection. Posttranslational modifications of proteins include phosphorylation, acetylation, AMPylation, ubiquitination, and ubiquitin-like modifications. Co-opting posttranslational modifications are emerging as a common strategy employed by pathogens to downregulate host responses (Randow and Lehner, 2009; Ribet and Cossart, 2010; Rytkonen and Holden, 2007), and many posttranslational modifications probably participate in the host cell response to *Listeria* infection.

A recent study has revealed that *Listeria* interferes with the host SUMOylation machinery (Ribet *et al.*, 2010). SUMOylation is a fundamental eukaryotic posttranslational modification involved in several key processes, including transcriptional regulation, intracellular transport, stress responses, and the maintenance of genome integrity (Kerscher *et al.*, 2006). Similar to the ubiquitin system, the conjugation of SUMO on to a lysine residue of a target protein involves an E1, E2, and E3 enzyme. Strikingly, LLO triggers degradation of Ubc9, the unique human E2 SUMO enzyme, and leads to a global decrease in the levels of SUMO-conjugated host proteins in host cells. SUMO overexpression counteracts infection, showing that *Listeria* decreases the SUMOylation level of proteins for efficient infection.

Interestingly, some listerial proteins are also posttranslationally modified by the host. For example, ActA is phosphorylated (Brundage *et al.*, 1993), and LLO is ubiquitinated (Schnupf *et al.*, 2006). Yet, the precise role of these modifications during infection *in vivo* is not yet known.

3.4. Gene reprogramming: Histone modifications and chromatin remodeling

L. monocytogenes is known to reprogram host genes during infection (reviewed in Cossart, in press), and recent discoveries studying host epigenetics have highlighted yet another strategy used by *Listeria* to reprogram gene expression. The transcriptional status of a gene is tightly linked to the structure of chromatin, and transcriptional regulation can be achieved via various epigenetic mechanisms. At the center of these mechanisms are histones and nucleosomes, the basic unit of chromatin. The NH_2 termini of the four core histones (H2A, H2B, H3, and H4) protrude out of the nucleosome, making them available for a variety of covalent posttranslational modifications, including phosphorylation, acetylation, methylation, and ubiquitination. The combination of different histone modifications account for the ''histone code'' that generates specific docking sites for proteins regulating chromatin structure and gene transcription, adding an additional level of regulation aside from regulation by activators or repressors which bind to defined sequences in the promoter region. Histone modifications and chromatin structure remodeling are key regulators of eukaryotic transcription and may therefore be potent targets for pathogens during infection (Hamon and Cossart, 2007).

Recent reports have shown that *L. monocytogenes* is able to induce histone modifications and chromatin remodeling, thereby inducing a specific transcriptional profile. LLO, and other toxins of the same family produced by extracellular pathogens, induces histone H3 dephosphorylation and H4 deacetylation early during infection and these events correlate with the downregulation of some immunity genes (Hamon and Cossart, 2007). LLO can induce these modifications from outside of the cell, showing that LLO can transcriptionally reprogram cells that are not infected. This phenomenon is dependent on LLO-induced K^+ efflux and is independent of caspase-1 activation (Hamon and Cossart, 2011). LLO-independent histone modifications have also been suggested (Hamon and Cossart, 2007), though how exactly these modifications are induced has not yet been deciphered. LntA is another *Listeria* virulence factor shown to affect chromatin (Lebreton *et al.*, 2011). LntA interacts with BAHD1, a protein which is part of a multiprotein complex involved in heterochromatin formation and gene silencing. Strikingly, LntA interacts with BAHD1 in the nucleus and induces expression of type III interferon genes and interferon-regulated genes (ISGs), and therefore manipulates the innate immune response. Together, these reports suggest that genes involved in inflammation and immunity can be regulated by *Listeria* via different epigenetic mechanisms. The diversity of mechanisms involved, and how important this phenomenon is *in vivo*, has yet to be determined.

4. CONCLUSIONS AND PERSPECTIVES

Over the past two decades, fundamental questions of cell biology have been productively addressed by using *Listeria* as a cellular tool. Conversely, cell biology approaches have revolutionized our view of *Listeria* pathogenesis. It is clear that the pathogenesis field has progressively shifted from the study of the mechanics of infection toward a better understanding of how pathogens co-opt host signaling cascades to modify the host transcriptional program and dampen the innate immune response. An important challenge now is to validate the concepts established in tissue culture cells at the single cell level *in vivo* in relevant animal models.

REFERENCES

Aubry, C., Goulard, C., Nahori, M.-A., Cayet, N., Decalf, J., Sachse, M., Boneca, I. G., Cossart, P., and Dussurget, O. (2011). OatA, a peptidoglycan O-acetyltransferase involved in *Listeria monocytogenes* immune escape, is critical for virulence. *J. Infect. Dis.* **204,** 731–740.

Bierne, H., and Cossart, P. (2002). InlB, a surface protein of *Listeria monocytogenes* that behaves as an invasin and a growth factor. *J. Cell Sci.* **115,** 3357–3367.

Bierne, H., and Cossart, P. (2007). *Listeria monocytogenes* surface proteins: From genome predictions to function. *Microbiol. Mol. Biol. Rev.* **71,** 377–397.

Birmingham, C. L., Canadien, V., Gouin, E., Troy, E. B., Yoshimori, T., Cossart, P., Higgins, D. E., and Brumell, J. H. (2007). *Listeria monocytogenes* evades killing by autophagy during colonization of host cells. *Autophagy* **3,** 442–451.

Birmingham, C. L., Canadien, V., Kaniuk, N. A., Steinberg, B. E., Higgins, D. E., and Brumell, J. H. (2008). Listeriolysin O allows *Listeria monocytogenes* replication in macrophage vacuoles. *Nature* **451,** 350–354.

Bonazzi, M., Vasudevan, L., Mallet, A., Sachse, M., Sartori, A., Prevost, M. C., Roberts, A., Taner, S. B., Wilbur, J. D., Brodsky, F. M., and Cossart, P. (2011). Clathrin phosphorylation is required for actin recruitment at sites of bacterial adhesion and internalization. *J. Cell Biol.* **195,** 525–536.

Boneca, I. G., Dussurget, O., Cabanes, D., Nahori, M.-A., Sousa, S., Lecuit, M., Psylinakis, E., Bouriotis, V., Hugot, J.-P., Giovannini, M., *et al.* (2007). A critical role for peptidoglycan N-deacetylation in *Listeria* evasion from the host innate immune system. *Proc. Natl. Acad. Sci. USA* **104,** 997–1002.

Boulant, S., Kural, C., Zeeh, J.-C., Ubelmann, F., and Kirchhausen, T. (2011). Actin dynamics counteract membrane tension during clathrin-mediated endocytosis. *Nat. Cell Biol.* **13,** 1124–1131.

Braun, L., Ghebrehiwet, B., and Cossart, P. (2000). gC1q-R/p32, a C1q-binding protein, is a receptor for the InlB invasion protein of *Listeria monocytogenes. EMBO J.* **19,** 1458–1466.

Brundage, R. A., Smith, G. A., Camilli, A., Theriot, J. A., and Portnoy, D. A. (1993). Expression and phosphorylation of the *Listeria monocytogenes* ActA protein in mammalian cells. *Proc. Natl. Acad. Sci. USA* **90,** 11890–11894.

Cameron, L. A., Footer, M. J., van Oudenaarden, A., and Theriot, J. A. (1999). Motility of ActA protein-coated microspheres driven by actin polymerization. *Proc. Natl. Acad. Sci. USA* **96,** 4908–4913.

Collins, A., Warrington, A., Taylor, Kenneth A., and Svitkina, T. (2011). Structural organization of the actin cytoskeleton at sites of clathrin-mediated endocytosis. *Curr. Biol.* **21,** 1167–1175.

Conner, S. D., and Schmid, S. L. (2003). Regulated portals of entry into the cell. *Nature* **422,** 37–44.

Cossart, P. (in press). Illuminating the landscape of host-pathogen interactions with *Listeria monocytogenes. Proc. Natl. Acad. Sci. USA.*

Cossart, P., Pizarro-Cerda, J., and Lecuit, M. (2003). Invasion of mammalian cells by *Listeria monocytogenes*: Functional mimicry to subvert cellular functions. *Trends Cell Biol.* **13,** 23–31.

Dortet, L., Mostowy, S., Samba Louaka, A., Gouin, E., Nahori, M. A., Weimer, E. A. C., Dussurget, O., and Cossart, P. (2011). Recruitment of the major vault protein: A *Listeria monocytogenes* strategy to avoid autophagy. *PLoS Pathog.* **7**(8), e1002168.

Fotin, A., Cheng, Y., Grigorieff, N., Walz, T., Harrison, S. C., and Kirchhausen, T. (2004). Structure of an auxilin-bound clathrin coat and its implications for the mechanism of uncoating. *Nature* **432,** 649–653.

Gouin, E., Welch, M. D., and Cossart, P. (2005). Actin-based motility of intracellular pathogens. *Curr. Opin. Microbiol.* **8,** 35–45.

Gouin, E., Adib-Conquy, M., Balestrino, D., Nahori, M. A., Villiers, V., Colland, F., Dramsi, S., Dussurget, O., and Cossart, P. (2010). The *Listeria monocytogenes* InlC protein interferes with innate immune responses by targeting the I{kappa}B kinase subunit IKK {alpha}. *Proc. Natl. Acad. Sci. USA* **107,** 17333–17338.

Green, D. R., Galluzzi, L., and Kroemer, G. (2011). Mitochondria and the autophagy-inflammation-cell death axis in organismal aging. *Science* **333,** 1109–1112.

Hall, P. A., and Russell, H. S. E. (2004). The pathobiology of the septin gene family. *J. Pathol.* **204,** 489–505.

Hamon, M., and Cossart, P. (2007). Histone modifications and chromatin remodeling during bacterial infections. *Cell Host Microbe* **1,** 100–109.

Hamon, M. A., and Cossart, P. (2011). K+ efflux, is required for histone-H3 dephosphorylation by Listeria LLO and other pore forming toxins. *Infect. Immun.* **79,** 2839–2846.

Hamon, M., Bierne, H., and Cossart, P. (2006). *Listeria monocytogenes*: A multifaceted model. *Nat. Rev. Microbiol.* **4,** 423–434.

He, C., and Klionsky, D. J. (2009). Regulation mechanisms and signaling pathways of autophagy. *Annu. Rev. Genet.* **43,** 67–93.

Huang, Y.-W., Yan, M., Collins, R. F., DiCiccio, J. E., Grinstein, S., and Trimble, W. S. (2008). Mammalian septins are required for phagosome formation. *Mol. Biol. Cell* **19,** 1717–1726.

John, C. M., Hite, R. K., Weirich, C. S., Fitzgerald, D. J., Jawhari, H., Faty, M., Schlapfer, D., Kroschewski, R., Winkler, F. K., Walz, T., *et al.* (2007). The *Caenorhabditis elegans* septin complex is nonpolar. *EMBO J.* **26,** 3296–3307.

Jonquières, R., Pizarro-Cerdá, J., and Cossart, P. (2001). Synergy between the N- and C-terminal domains of InlB for efficient invasion of non-phagocytic cells by *Listeria monocytogenes*. *Mol. Microbiol.* **42,** 955–965.

Kathryn, A. R., Chelsea, B., and Paul, W. (2003). Cytoplasmic bacteria can be targets for autophagy. *Cell. Microbiol.* **5,** 455–468.

Kerscher, O., Felberbaum, R., and Hochstrasser, M. (2006). Modification of proteins by ubiquitin and ubiquitin-like proteins. *Annu. Rev. Cell Dev. Biol.* **22,** 159–180.

Kinoshita, M. (2003). The septins. *Genome Biol.* **4,** 236.

Kocks, C., Hellio, R., Gounon, P., Ohayon, H., and Cossart, P. (1993). Polarized distribution of *Listeria monocytogenes* surface protein ActA at the site of directional actin assembly. *J. Cell Sci.* **105,** 699–710.

Lebreton, A., Lakisic, G., Job, V., Fritsch, L., Tham, T. N., Camejo, A., Mattei, P.-J., Regnault, B., Nahori, M. A., Cabanes, D., *et al.* (2011). A bacterial protein targets the BAHD1 chromatin complex to stimulate type III interferon response. *Science* **331,** 1319–1321.

Levine, B., and Deretic, V. (2007). Unveiling the roles of autophagy in innate and adaptive immunity. *Nat. Rev. Immunol.* **7,** 767–777.

Levine, B., and Klionsky, D. J. (2004). Development by self-digestion. *Dev. Cell* **6,** 463–477.

Levine, B., and Kroemer, G. (2008). Autophagy in the pathogenesis of disease. *Cell* **132,** 27–42.

Levine, B., Mizushima, N., and Virgin, H. W. (2011). Autophagy in immunity and inflammation. *Nature* **469,** 323–335.

Loisel, T. P., Boujemaa, R., Pantaloni, D., and Carlier, M.-F. (1999). Reconstitution of actin-based motility of *Listeria* and *Shigella* using pure proteins. *Nature* **401,** 613–616.

Mengaud, J., Ohayon, H., Gounon, P., Mège, R.-M., and Cossart, P. (1996). E-cadherin is the receptor for internalin, a surface protein required for entry of *L. monocytogenes* into epithelial cells. *Cell* **84,** 923–932.

Mizushima, N., Levine, B., Cuervo, A. M., and Klionsky, D. J. (2008). Autophagy fights disease through cellular self-digestion. *Nature* **451,** 1069–1075.

Mostowy, S., Danckaert, A., Tham, T. N., Machu, C., Guadagnini, S., Pizarro-Cerda, J., and Cossart, P. (2009a). Septin 11 restricts InlB-mediated invasion by *Listeria*. *J. Biol. Chem.* **284,** 11613–11621.

Mostowy, S., Nam Tham, T., Danckaert, A., Guadagnini, S., Boisson-Dupuis, S., Pizarro-Cerda, J., and Cossart, P. (2009b). Septins regulate bacterial entry into host cells. *PLoS One* **4,** e4196.

Mostowy, S., Bonazzi, M., Hamon, M., Tham, T. N., Mallet, A., Lelek, M., Gouin, E., Demangel, C., Brosch, R., Zimmer, C., *et al.* (2010). Entrapment of intracytosolic bacteria by septin cage-like structures. *Cell Host Microbe* **18,** 433–444.

Mostowy, S., Janel, S., Forestier, C., Roduit, C., Kasas, S., Pizarro-Cerda, J., Cossart, P., and Lafont, F. (2011a). A role for septins in the interaction between the *Listeria monocytogenes* invasion protein InlB and the Met receptor. *Biophys. J.* **100,** 1949–1959.

Mostowy, S., Sancho-Shimizu, V., Hamon, M., Simeone, R., Brosch, R., Johansen, T., and Cossart, P. (2011b). p62 and NDP52 proteins target intracytosolic *Shigella* and *Listeria* to different autophagy pathways. *J. Biol. Chem.* **286,** 26987–26995.

Pankiv, S., Clausen, T. H., Lamark, T., Brech, A., Bruun, J.-A., Outzen, H., Øvervatn, A., Bjørkøy, G., and Johansen, T. (2007). p62/SQSTM1 binds directly to Atg8/LC3 to facilitate degradation of ubiquitinated protein aggregates by autophagy. *J. Biol. Chem.* **282,** 24131–24145.

Perrin, A. J., Jiang, X., Birmingham, C. L., So, N. S. Y., and Brumell, J. H. (2004). Recognition of bacteria in the cytosol of mammalian cells by the ubiquitin system. *Curr. Biol.* **14,** 806–811.

Pizarro-Cerda, J., and Cossart, P. (2006). Bacterial adhesion and entry into host cells. *Cell* **124,** 715–727.

Pizarro-Cerda, J., and Cossart, P. (2009). *Listeria monocytogenes* membrane trafficking and lifestyle: The exception or the rule? *Annu. Rev. Cell Dev. Biol.* **25,** 649–670.

Radtke, A. L., Anderson, K. L., Davis, M. J., DiMagno, M. J., Swanson, J. A., and O'Riordan, M. X. (2011). *Listeria monocytogenes* exploits cystic fibrosis transmembrane conductance regulator (CFTR) to escape the phagosome. *Proc. Natl. Acad. Sci. USA* **108,** 1633–1638.

Rae, C. S., Geissler, A., Adamson, P. C., and Portnoy, D. A. (2011). Mutations of the *Listeria monocytogenes* peptidoglycan N-deacetylase and O-acetylase result in enhanced lysozyme sensitivity, bacteriolysis, and hyperinduction of innate immune pathways. *Infect. Immun.* **79,** 3596–3606.

Rajabian, T., Gavicherla, B., Heisig, M., Muller-Altrock, S., Goebel, W., Gray-Owen, S. D., and Ireton, K. (2009). The bacterial virulence factor InlC perturbs apical cell junctions and promotes cell-to-cell spread of *Listeria*. *Nat. Cell Biol.* **11,** 1212–1218.

Randow, F., and Lehner, P. J. (2009). Viral avoidance and exploitation of the ubiquitin system. *Nat. Cell Biol.* **11,** 527–534.

Ribet, D., and Cossart, P. (2010). Pathogen-mediated posttranslational modifications: A re-emerging field. *Cell* **143,** 694–702.

Ribet, D., Hamon, M., Gouin, E., Nahori, M.-A., Impens, F., Neyret-Kahn, H., Gevaert, K., Vandekerckhove, J., Dejean, A., and Cossart, P. (2010). Listeria monocytogenes impairs sumoylation for efficient infection. *Nature* **464,** 1192–1195.

Robbins, J. R., Barth, A. I., Marquis, H., de Hostos, E. L., Nelson, W. J., and Theriot, J. A. (1999). *Listeria monocytogenes* exploits normal host cell processes to spread from cell to cell. *J. Cell Biol.* **146,** 1333–1350.

Rubinsztein, D. C. (2006). The roles of intracellular protein-degradation pathways in neurodegeneration. *Nature* **443,** 780–786.

Rudel, T., Kepp, O., and Kozjak-Pavlovic, V. (2010). Interactions between bacterial pathogens and mitochondrial cell death pathways. *Nat. Rev. Microbiol.* **8,** 693–705.

Rytkonen, A., and Holden, D. W. (2007). Bacterial interference of ubiquitination and deubiquitination. *Cell Host Microbe* **1,** 13–22.

Saarikangas, J., and Barral, Y. (2011). The emerging functions of septins in metazoans. *EMBO Rep.* **12,** 118–126.

Sandrock, K., Bartsch, I., Blaser, S., Busse, A., Busse, E., and Zieger, B. (2011). Characterization of human septin interactions. *Biol. Chem.* **392,** 751–761.

Schnupf, P., and Portnoy, D. A. (2007). Listeriolysin O: A phagosome-specific lysin. *Microbes Infect.* **9,** 1176–1187.

Schnupf, P., Portnoy, D. A., and Decatur, A. L. (2006). Phosphorylation, ubiquitination and degradation of listeriolysin O in mammalian cells: Role of the PEST-like sequence. *Cell. Microbiol.* **8,** 353–364.

Sellin, M. E., Sandblad, L., Stenmark, S., and Gullberg, M. (2011). Deciphering the rules governing assembly order of mammalian septin complexes. *Mol. Biol. Cell* **22,** 3152–3164.

Shaughnessy, L. M., Adam, D. H., Kenneth, A. C., and Joel, A. S. (2006). Membrane perforations inhibit lysosome fusion by altering pH and calcium in *Listeria monocytogenes* vacuoles. *Cell. Microbiol.* **8,** 781–792.

Shen, Y., Naujokas, M., Park, M., and Ireton, K. (2000). InlB-dependent internalization of *Listeria* is mediated by the Met receptor tyrosine kinase. *Cell* **103,** 501–510.

Shintani, T., and Klionsky, D. J. (2004). Autophagy in health and disease: A double-edged sword. *Science* **306,** 990–995.

Singh, R., Jamieson, A., and Cresswell, P. (2008). GILT is a critical host factor for *Listeria monocytogenes* infection. *Nature* **455,** 1244–1247.

Sirajuddin, M., Farkasovsky, M., Hauer, F., Kuhlmann, D., Macara, I. G., Weyand, M., Stark, H., and Wittinghofer, A. (2007). Structural insight into filament formation by mammalian septins. *Nature* **449,** 311–315.

Smith, G. A., Marquis, H., Jones, S., Johnston, N. C., Portnoy, D. A., and Goldfine, H. (1995). The two distinct phospholipases C of *Listeria monocytogenes* have overlapping roles in escape from a vacuole and cell-to-cell spread. *Infect. Immun.* **63,** 4231–4237.

Sorkin, A. (2004). Cargo recognition during clathrin-mediated endocytosis: A team effort. *Curr. Opin. Cell Biol.* **16,** 392–399.

Spiliotis, E. T., and Gladfelter, A. S. (2011). Spatial guidance of cell asymmetry: Septin GTPases show the way. *Traffic.*

Stavru, F., Archambaud, C., and Cossart, P. (2011a). Cell biology and immunology of *Listeria monocytogenes* infections: Novel insights. *Immunol. Rev.* **240,** 160–184.

Stavru, F., Bouillaud, F., Sartori, A., Ricquier, D., and Cossart, P. (2011b). *Listeria monocytogenes* transiently alters mitochondrial dynamics during infection. *Proc. Natl. Acad. Sci. USA* **108,** 3612–3617.

Thurston, T. L. M., Ryzhakov, G., Bloor, S., von Muhlinen, N., and Randow, F. (2009). The TBK1 adaptor and autophagy receptor NDP52 restricts the proliferation of ubiquitin-coated bacteria. *Nat. Immunol.* **10,** 1215–1221.

Van Troys, M., Lambrechts, A., David, V., Demol, H., Puype, M., Pizarro-Cerda, J., Gevaert, K., Cossart, P., and Vandekerckhove, J. (2008). The actin propulsive machinery: The proteome of *Listeria monocytogenes* tails. *Biochem. Biophys. Res. Commun.* **375,** 194–199.

Vazquez-Boland, J. A., Kocks, C., Dramsi, S., Ohayon, H., Geoffroy, C., Mengaud, J., and Cossart, P. (1992). Nucleotide sequence of the lecithinase operon of *Listeria monocytogenes* and possible role of lecithinase in cell-to-cell spread. *Infect. Immun.* **60,** 219–230.

Veiga, E., and Cossart, P. (2005). *Listeria* hijacks the clathrin-dependent endocytic machinery to invade mammalian cells. *Nat. Cell Biol.* **7,** 894–900.

Veiga, E., Guttman, J. A., Bonazzi, M., Boucrot, E., Toledo-Arana, A., Lin, A. E., Enninga, J., Pizarro-Cerda, J., Finlay, B. B., Kirchhausen, T., *et al.* (2007). Invasive and adherent bacterial pathogens co-opt host clathrin for infection. *Cell Host Microbe* **2,** 340–351.

Vellai, T., Takács-Vellai, K., Sass, M., and Klionsky, D. J. (2009). The regulation of aging: Does autophagy underlie longevity? *Trends Cell Biol.* **19,** 487–494.

Weirich, C. S., Erzberger, J. P., and Barral, Y. (2008). The septin family of GTPases: Architecture and dynamics. *Nat. Rev. Mol. Cell Biol.* **9,** 478–489.

Welch, M. D., Iwamatsu, A., and Mitchison, T. J. (1997). Actin polymerization is induced by Arp 2/3 protein complex at the surface of *Listeria monocytogenes*. *Nature* **385,** 265–269.

West, A. P., Shadel, G. S., and Ghosh, S. (2011). Mitochondria in innate immune responses. *Nat. Rev. Immunol.* **11,** 389–402.

Wild, P., Farhan, H., McEwan, D. G., Wagner, S., Rogov, V. V., Brady, N. R., Richter, B., Korac, J., Waidmann, O., Choudhary, C., *et al.* (2011). Phosphorylation of the autophagy receptor optineurin restricts *Salmonella* growth. *Science* **333,** 228–233.

Yoshikawa, Y., Ogawa, M., Hain, T., Yoshida, M., Fukumatsu, M., Kim, M., Mimuro, H., Nakagawa, I., Yanagawa, T., Ishii, T., *et al.* (2009). *Listeria monocytogenes* ActA-mediated escape from autophagic recognition. *Nat. Cell Biol.* **11,** 1233–1240.

CHAPTER 4

Dendritic Cells in *Listeria monocytogenes* Infection

Brian T. Edelson

Contents

Abstract

Dendritic cells (DCs) represent a unique collection of innate immune cells present throughout the body as distinct subpopulations generally sharing the functions of pathogen recognition, cytokine production, and antigen presentation. A large body of work in recent years has examined DC functions during infection with *Listeria monocytogenes* (Lm), particularly in the murine model. Here, I review several aspects of DC biology in this model, with

Department of Pathology and Immunology, Washington University School of Medicine, St. Louis, Missouri, USA

Advances in Immunology, Volume 113
ISSN 0065-2776, DOI: 10.1016/B978-0-12-394590-7.00006-3

particular emphasis on the role DCs play in the establishment of a productive Lm infection and the role of DCs as cytokine producers and antigen-presenting cells in this system.

1. INTRODUCTION

Systemic infection of mice with *Listeria monocytogenes* (Lm) has proven to be a very useful model for dissection of the immune response to this Gram-positive intracellular bacterium (Stavru *et al.*, 2011). Inoculation by either the intraperitoneal or the intravenous routes results in infection largely confined to the spleen and liver, although other organs including peripheral lymph nodes (Solodova *et al.*, 2011), the gallbladder (Hardy *et al.*, 2004), the brain (Berche, 1995), and the fetoplacental unit during pregnancy (Disson *et al.*, 2008) can be infected. An array of virulence factors are used by Lm to survive within the host environment, chief amongst them listeriolysin O (LLO), which allows the bacterium access to the host cell cytosol (Stavru *et al.*, 2011). Professional phagocytes, including dendritic cells (DCs), macrophages, monocytes, and neutrophils (Aoshi *et al.*, 2009), all trap circulating bacteria quickly within infected organs and, upon sensing infection, coordinate an initial inflammatory response aimed at control of bacterial growth. This initial response includes the production of numerous cytokines and chemokines, and involves migration and activation of natural killer (NK) cells and monocytes which together result in interferon-γ (IFN-γ), tumor necrosis factor (TNF), and nitric oxide production (Kang *et al.*, 2008). If these mechanisms are in place, and initial Lm load is not overwhelming, bacterial burden can be controlled for the first 3–4 days of infection, allowing the priming of Lm-specific CD4 and CD8 T cell responses. These cells eradicate the pathogen over days 4–10 of infection and provide long-lived T cell memory. This review will focus on the role of DCs in the mouse model of Lm infection, as they are key participants in all stages of the immune response to this organism. I will initially provide a brief introduction to DC biology.

1.1. DC development

DCs represent a collection of mononuclear phagocytes present in both lymphoid and nonlymphoid organs, distinct from monocytes and macrophages. Several recent reviews have described their development and categorization in the murine system (Geissmann *et al.*, 2010a,b; Liu and Nussenzweig, 2010). As a group, mouse DCs all express the integrin CD11c (integrin α_X) and MHC class II (both of which can also be expressed at times on monocytes or macrophages), but are classified as subsets based on their expression of a variety of other cell surface markers. They are bone marrow derived, developing from a committed DC progenitor termed the common-DC progenitor (CDP) (Naik *et al.*, 2007; Onai *et al.*, 2007). CDPs themselves develop from a less differentiated precursor cell that has the capacity to generate monocytes, macrophages, and DCs, termed the macrophage-DC progenitor (MDP) (Fogg *et al.*, 2006). The MDP is derived from the common myeloid progenitor (CMP). CDPs in the bone marrow develop into both plasmacytoid DCs (pDCs), a DC subset whose specialized function is the rapid production of type I IFN upon viral infection, and pre-DCs, which leave the bone marrow and migrate via the blood to lymphoid and nonlymphoid tissues as precursors of conventional DCs (cDCs).

1.2. DC subsets

cDCs of lymphoid organs are divided into two subsets, both of which are highly efficient at pathogen detection and antigen presentation. These subsets are unique in terms of their gene expression patterns (Dudziak *et al.*, 2007) and therefore are functionally specialized in terms of their antigen processing pathways, pathogen recognition systems, and cytokine responses. Several transcription factors control the development of these subsets, such that mice deficient in these factors fail to develop one or more DC subsets (Geissmann *et al.*, 2010b). In the mouse, $CD8\alpha^+$ DCs are highly efficient at antigen cross-presentation, a process whereby exogenous proteins derived from the phagocytic pathway, sometimes coming from dead or dying cells, are processed and presented on MHC class I molecules to CD8 T cells (Lin *et al.*, 2008). $CD8\alpha^-$ DCs are more efficient at processing proteins for presentation by MHC class II molecules to CD4 T cells (Dudziak *et al.*, 2007). The marker CD8α only allows DC subset discrimination in mouse lymphoid tissues, but a similar division of human DCs subsets has recently been revealed (Bachem *et al.*, 2010; Crozat *et al.*, 2010; Jongbloed *et al.*, 2010; Poulin *et al.*, 2010), with the markers CD141 (BDCA3), CLEC9A (DNGR1), and XCR1 all marking a population of human DCs sharing with mouse $CD8\alpha^+$ DCs the properties of TLR3 expression, IL-12 production, dead cell uptake, and cross-presentation.

Nonlymphoid tissue DCs have largely been studied in the skin, lung, and intestinal lamina propria, although they are also described in the liver, pancreas, kidney, and brain (Helft *et al.*, 2010). These DCs migrate through afferent lymphatics to tissue draining lymph nodes, in both the steady state and during inflammation, where they can prime T cell responses. In most of these organs, two subsets exist, marked as either $CD103^+CD11b^{low/-}$ or $CD103^-CD11b^+$ DCs. $CD103^+CD11b^{low/-}$ DCs as a group appear closely related to $CD8\alpha^+$ DCs of the lymphoid tissue, based on their gene expression, function, developmental requirements for transcription factors, and precursor cell of origin, the pre-DC. Peripheral $CD103^-CD11b^+$ DCs, on the other hand, appear to develop from both pre-DCs and monocytes in the steady state. Certain tissues also contain unique subsets of DCs that do not fit the simple dichotomy of $CD103^+CD11b^{low/-}$ and $CD103^-CD11b^+$ DCs, including Langerhans cells of the epidermis, and $CD103^+CD11b^+$ DCs of the lamina propria. The study of peripheral tissue DC function is an active area of investigation, and likely these DCs play important roles during bacterial infections outside the lymphoid tissue.

1.3. Monocyte-derived DCs

One last form of DC that deserves mention here is the inflammation-driven blood monocyte-derived DC, sometimes referred to as the inflammatory monocyte or the inflammatory DC (Serbina *et al.*, 2008). This form of DC arises in settings of infection or autoimmunity and shares expression of typical DC markers with cDCs (e.g., CD11c and MHC class II). In addition, these DCs are able to prime T cell responses, a function typically thought of as unique to DCs. Inflammatory DCs develop from activated $Ly6C^+$ monocytes, usually in settings of TLR engagement and IFN-γ stimulation. The prototypical inflammatory DC is the so-called TNF- and inducible nitric oxide synthase (iNOS)-producing DC (Tip-DC) first described in the mouse spleen during the early phase of Lm infection (Serbina *et al.*, 2003). *In vitro*, bone marrow cells or purified monocytes cultured with granulocyte-macrophage colony stimulating factor (GM-CSF) differentiate into cells displaying the hallmark features of Tip-DCs (Xu *et al.*, 2007). GM-CSF-receptor deficient mice, however, retain the ability to generate Tip-DCs upon Lm infection (Brian T. Edelson, unpublished data), suggesting that other monocyte activating signals lead to Tip-DC differentiation *in vivo* in the absence of GM-CSF signaling. Nevertheless, a number of studies have examined the interaction between GM-CSF-derived DCs and Lm, likely better representing Tip-DCs in this regard. A separate chapter in this issue of *Advances in Immunology* will focus on monocytes and Lm, and therefore the scope of my review will be limited to the roles of cDCs and pDCs during Lm infection.

2. DCS IN ESTABLISHMENT OF LM INFECTION

2.1. Splenic architecture

The mouse spleen consists of lymphoid sheaths surrounding central arterioles (seen as white pulp follicles on cross section), coursing through areas of red pulp, where venous sinuses collect blood for return to the circulation (Mebius and Kraal, 2005). White pulp follicles contain an inner sheath of T cells, the so-called periarteriolar lymphoid sheath (PALS), and an outer sheath of B cells. Separating this B cell area from the red pulp is the marginal zone, an important location for trapping of blood-borne pathogens. The marginal zone contains two distinct resident macrophage subsets, as well as DCs and specialized marginal zone B cells. Initial histologic studies of Lm infection of the mouse revealed phagocytosed bacteria within splenic macrophages (Armstrong and Sword, 1966) and significant T cell depletion in the PALS beginning at day 1 after infection (Chan and Cheers, 1982). This T cell depletion was later recognized to involve apoptosis (Merrick *et al.*, 1997). The earliest events taking place in the Lm-infected spleen, however, were first examined histologically by Conlan (1996), who identified initial Lm uptake by morphologically distinct macrophages and DCs within the marginal zone as early as 1 h after infection. By 12 h, these same infected phagocytes were seen within the white pulp, and by 24 h neutrophils were extensively infiltrating the white pulp and also contained bacteria.

2.2. Splenic DC infection by Lm

Whether Lm transport to the PALS was an important aspect of productive splenic infection and whether DCs were required for this transport remained unanswered questions, although a series of observations began to focus attention on DCs in this process. Mice treated with Flt3 ligand (Flt3L) showed expansion of both CD8α^+ and CD8α^- DCs in the spleen and showed increased Lm burden early after infection (Alaniz *et al.*, 2004). The next major breakthrough came with the surprising realization that CD11c-diptheria toxin receptor (DTR) transgenic mice transiently depleted of CD11c-expressing cells were markedly resistant to splenic Lm infection (Neuenhahn *et al.*, 2006). Diptheria toxin treatment of these mice is known to deplete both DCs and radioresistant splenic macrophages, but infection experiments in radiation chimeras proved that DC depletion was responsible for the resistance to Lm. Similarly, Lm resistance was observed in CD11c-cre × ROSA26-flox-stop-flox-diptheria toxin A (DTA) mice, a model of constitutive DC deficiency (Kang *et al.*, 2008). Cell sorting experiments revealed that CD8α^+ DCs were preferentially infected with Lm on a per cell basis in the first few hours of infection, before bacteria spread to CD8α^- DCs, monocytes, macrophages, and neutrophils (Neuenhahn *et al.*, 2006). These sorting experiments, however, were probably unable to appreciate the full spectrum of early macrophage Lm uptake, as marginal zone macrophages and marginal zone metallophilic macrophages are not readily amenable to extraction upon collagenase digestion. A broader uptake of Lm by DCs, red pulp macrophages, marginal zone macrophages, and marginal zone metallophilic macrophages was revealed by immunostaining experiments early after infection (Aoshi *et al.*, 2009), with most of this trapping occurring within the marginal zone. Within the past year, other groups have used either flow cytometry with GFP- or CFSE-labeled Lm or a cell sorting strategy similar to Neuenhahn *et al.* to confirm early infection of $CD8\alpha^+$ DCs (Campisi *et al.*, 2011; Lyszkiewicz *et al.*, 2011; Mitchell *et al.*, 2011; Zhan *et al.*, 2011), although specific proof of an absolute requirement for $CD8\alpha^+$ DCs in establishment of Lm infection has been lacking until very recently (see below).

Other observations are relevant here. Both CD11c-DTR mice depleted of DCs and mice treated with clodronate liposomes to deplete DCs showed reduced movement of Lm from the marginal zone to the PALS (Aoshi *et al.*, 2008), although both of these experiments have the caveat that these DC depletion strategies also affect splenic macrophages. Treatment of mice with pertussis toxin, to inhibit cell migration via chemokine receptors, also blocked Lm transport from the marginal zone to the PALS, consistent with this movement occurring within a migrating host cell (Aoshi *et al.*, 2008). Conversely, mice bearing DC-specific depletion of the lipid phosphatase Pten, and therefore displaying an expanded population of splenic $CD8\alpha^+$ DCs, showed increased susceptibility to Lm infection and increased bacteria within the PALS at 24 h after infection (Sathaliyawala *et al.*, 2010).

2.3. Splenic $CD8\alpha^+$ DC localization

Neuenhahn *et al.* used immunostaining to examine uninfected mouse spleens for the localization of $CD8\alpha^+$ DCs (Neuenhahn *et al.*, 2006). Previously, immunostaining of spleen sections for the surface marker CD205 (DEC205), expressed on all mouse $CD8\alpha^+$ DCs by flow cytometry, had shown $CD8\alpha^+$ DCs to localize selectively to the PALS (Kraal *et al.*, 1986). This location, however, seemed incongruent with the observation that $CD8\alpha^+$ DCs were rapidly infected with Lm, as this was thought to take place in the marginal zone. Neuenhahn *et al.* used costaining of $CD8\alpha$ and CD11c to identify $CD8\alpha^+$ DCs in spleen sections, rather than relying on CD205 staining, and found, in fact, that $CD8\alpha^+$ DCs were present within the marginal zone and red pulp, in addition to the PALS (Neuenhahn *et al.*, 2006). More recently, immunostaining of sections with an antibody to CD207 (Langerin), expressed within the spleen only on $CD8\alpha^+$ DCs, has confirmed that the majority of $CD8\alpha^+$ DCs are localized to the marginal zone in the steady state and that these DCs move to the PALS upon injection of the TLR agonists polyinosinic:polycytidylic acid (poly IC) or lipopolysaccharide (LPS) (Idoyaga *et al.*, 2009).

2.4. Splenic CD8α^+ DCs are required for Lm infection

Edelson *et al.* have now proven a specific requirement for CD8α^+ DCs in establishing Lm infection *in vivo*, using mice deficient in the transcription factor *Batf3* (Edelson *et al.*, 2011). These mice lack CD8α^+ DCs in lymphoid organs and CD103$^+$CD11b$^{low/-}$ DCs in peripheral tissues (Edelson *et al.*, 2010; Hildner *et al.*, 2008), but unlike other transcription factor-deficient mice which lack these DC subsets (i.e., *Irf8*$^{-/-}$, *Id2*$^{-/-}$, and *Nfil3*$^{-/-}$), *Batf3*$^{-/-}$ mice show no defects in other immune cell lineages. *Batf3*$^{-/-}$ mice, like pan-DC-depleted CD11c-DTR mice, are profoundly resistant to Lm infection, with $\sim$1/1000 of the bacterial burden in the spleen at day 3 after infection, and a significant increase in the median lethal dose (LD50). Absence of CD8α^+ DCs prevents movement of bacteria to the PALS, and in *Batf3*$^{-/-}$ mice, at 18 h Lm organisms colocalize with collections of neutrophils in the extrafollicular space. Interestingly, neutrophil depletion in *Batf3*$^{-/-}$ mice does not impact on their splenic Lm resistance (although it does result in a higher Lm burden in the liver), suggesting that mechanisms other than neutrophils exist for control of bacterial replication in the spleen if organisms are prevented from access to the PALS.

Edelson *et al.* also used anti-CD207 immunostaining to directly identify Lm-infected CD8α^+ DCs *in situ* (Edelson *et al.*, 2011). By 6 h after infection, most CD8α^+ DCs had migrated from the marginal zone to the PALS. Notably, however, only a small fraction of these DCs contained Lm. This movement of Lm-infected CD8α^+ DCs to the PALS was reminiscent of that observed after systemic injection of poly IC or LPS (Idoyaga *et al.*, 2009). In both of these systems, and after Lm injection, CD207 staining disappeared at later time points, suggesting either decreased expression of this marker, or cell death. Along these lines, Edelson *et al.* observed loss of CD8α^+ DCs from infected spleens by flow cytometry (using the markers CD8α and CD205), with the magnitude of this loss correlating with inoculum size. Others have also observed a loss of DCs during Lm infection (Mitchell *et al.*, 2011; Muraille *et al.*, 2007), suggesting the hypothesis that Lm induces death of these cells, either directly or indirectly. A model for early Lm infection of the mouse spleen is presented in Fig. 4.1.

It is important to consider why infection of a small number of CD8α^+ DCs is so critical to the explosive Lm replication that occurs upon transport to the PALS. Whether CD8α^+ DCs are particularly permissive to Lm infection, compared to the other phagocytes which also initially participate in uptake of Lm, is an open question, although *ex vivo* data suggest that this may be the case (Kapadia *et al.*, 2011). Likewise, cells of the PALS, perhaps tingible-body macrophages, or other stromal components, may be permissive for Lm replication and serve as the site for this stage of infection after CD8α^+ DC-mediated delivery. It is also possible that

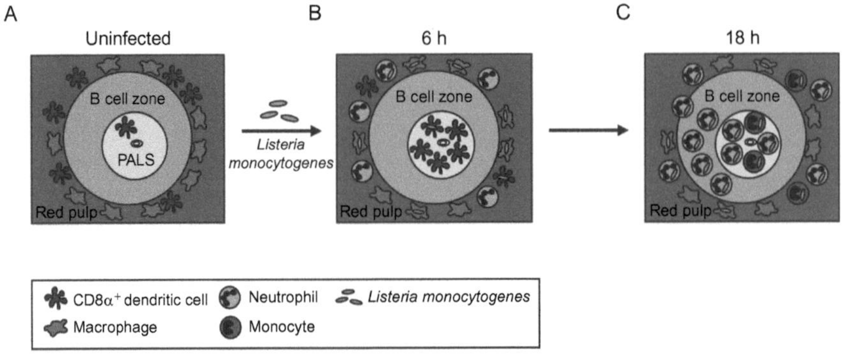

FIGURE 4.1 Model of splenic Lm infection. (A) In the uninfected mouse spleen, CD8α^+ DCs and marginal zone macrophages populate the marginal zone around white pulp follicles. Rare CD8α^+ DCs are also present in the PALS. (B) At 6 h after infection with Lm, bacteria are largely contained within macrophages of the marginal zone. CD8α^+ DCs have largely moved to the PALS, although these cells are only rarely infected. Neutrophils begin to infiltrate the spleen, but are present outside follicles. (C) At 18 h after infection, bacteria are largely contained within neutrophils, which have mostly infiltrated the follicles. Inflammatory monocytes have also begun to enter the follicle and contain intracellular bacteria. At high doses of infection, CD8α^+ DCs are eliminated from the spleen. (See Color Insert.)

neutrophils or monocytes, although largely serving an antimicrobial function, may also be hosts for intracellular growth of Lm within the PALS, if these cells cannot completely block bacterial access to the cytosol.

2.5. Peripheral tissue DCs during Lm infection

The issue of whether DCs play roles in establishing Lm infection in peripheral tissues is particularly interesting. In the mouse liver, pDCs and cDCs are known to exist. As in other peripheral organs, hepatic cDCs can be divided into CD103$^+$CD11b$^{low/-}$ and CD103$^-$CD11b$^+$ subsets, although CD103$^-$CD11b$^-$ DCs are also present. *Batf3*$^{-/-}$, *Id2*$^{-/-}$, and *Irf8*-mutant mice all selectively lack CD103$^+$CD11b$^{low/-}$ hepatic DCs (Edelson *et al.*, 2010; Ginhoux *et al.*, 2009), confirming the developmental, and likely, functional similarity between this peripheral tissue DC subset and CD8α^+ DCs. Kupffer cells, the resident macrophages of the liver, are known to be responsible for the majority of Lm trapping following inoculation (Gregory *et al.*, 2002), although it is not known whether liver DCs also participate in this to some extent.

Batf3$^{-/-}$ mice are markedly resistant to Lm infection in both the liver and spleen, as early as day 1 of infection, suggesting a role for CD103$^+$CD11b$^{low/-}$ hepatic DCs in establishing liver infection (Edelson *et al.*, 2011). These mice also show resistance to *Listeria ivanovii*, a related *Listeria* species known to selectively infect the mouse liver, ruling out the hypothesis that liver resistance in these mice is simply a reflection of less splenic infection. Liver resistance to Lm infection was also reported in CD11c-cre × ROSA26-flox-stop-flox-DTA mice, although in this report quantitative data on organ Lm burden was not provided (Kang *et al.*, 2008). Notably, CD11c-DTR mice showed Lm resistance only in the spleen (Neuenhahn *et al.*, 2006). Conceivably, this could have been due to incomplete depletion of hepatic DCs (particularly $CD103^{+}CD11b^{low/-}$ DCs) upon treatment with diphtheria toxin, as incomplete depletion of peripheral $CD103^{+}$ DCs in CD11c-DTR mice has been reported in other tissues (Geurts van Kessel *et al.*, 2008). Nonetheless, the results in $Batf3^{-/-}$ mice and CD11c-cre × ROSA26-flox-stop-flox-DTA mice are compelling, and further experiments will be required to define precisely how hepatic DCs function during Lm infection.

Conceivably, oral Lm infection, the natural route of human Lm disease, may also involve DCs. An important role for the Lm virulence factor internalin A (InlA) in this process is clear, as this protein on the bacterial surface serves as a ligand for E-cadherin, expressed on intestinal epithelial cells. This interaction promotes internalization of the bacteria by these nonprofessional phagocytes (Lecuit *et al.*, 2001; Wollert *et al.*, 2007). Whether infection proceeds from the epithelial layer to the lamina propria by way of infecting DCs or whether spread from the intestine to the mesenteric lymph node (MLN) requires DCs is unknown. In a mouse model of *Salmonella* infection forced to occur by way of epithelial cell invasion (rather than through Peyer's patch uptake), $CD103^{+}CD11b^{+}$ DCs were responsible for transport to the MLN (Bogunovic *et al.*, 2009). In a ligated ileal loop model of oral Lm infection in the rat, Peyer's patch DCs (marked by the rat pan-DC marker OX-62 (CD103)) located below the epithelium were the first cells infected and delivered Lm to the MLN within 6 h (Pron *et al.*, 2001). It should be possible to specifically examine the role of $CD103^{+}CD11b^{low/-}$ intestinal DCs during oral Lm infection in $Batf3^{-/-}$ mice, as they selectively lack this subset (Edelson *et al.*, 2010).

3. DC CYTOKINE PRODUCTION DURING LM INFECTION

While blood monocyte-derived DCs clearly represent an important source of cytokines (particularly TNF) during Lm infection, few studies have carefully examined *in vivo* cytokine production by pDCs or cDCs during Lm infection. Here I will focus on two aspects of DC cytokine production, pDCs as nonproducers of type I interferon (IFN-I) during Lm infection and cDCs as producers of IL-12 during this response.

3.1. pDCs during Lm infection

pDCs are critical sources of type I IFN during diverse viral infections, through their sensing of viral nucleic acids via TLR7 and TLR9 (Swiecki and Colonna, 2010). In contrast to type I IFN's protective antiviral role, endogenous type I IFN produced during Lm infection results in increased susceptibility to Lm, such that mice deficient in the type I IFN receptor (IFNAR$^{-/-}$) are profoundly resistant to Lm infection (Auerbuch *et al.*, 2004; Carrero *et al.*, 2004; O'Connell *et al.*, 2004). Therefore, it became important to ask whether pDCs represented an important source of type I IFN after Lm infection. Three studies have examined this carefully. Stockinger *et al.* were the first to suggest that pDCs were, in fact, non-producers of type I IFN during early Lm infection, with the type I IFN producing cell instead bearing the surface markings of a CD11b^{+} splenic macrophage (Stockinger *et al.*, 2009). Dressing *et al.* used an IFNβ fluorescent reporter-knockin mouse to demonstrate that Tip-DCs were the source of IFNβ during Lm infection, with this response peaking at 24 h after infection and localizing to infected areas of white pulp (Dresing *et al.*, 2010). Most recently, Solodova *et al.* used a conditional IFNβ reporter mouse and also concluded that Tip-DCs were the major source of type I IFN and that IFNβ was the critical form of type I IFN mediating susceptibility to Lm infection (Solodova *et al.*, 2011). This study also showed that antibody-mediated depletion of pDCs with anti-PDCA-1 did not alter Lm resistance. A more specific model of pDC depletion using BDCA-2-DTR transgenic mice has confirmed no role of pDCs in affecting organ Lm burden (Swiecki and Colonna, 2010). Overall, these studies point out how different pathogen infections (i.e., viruses vs. intracellular bacteria) elicit type I IFN responses from different cell types.

3.2. IL-12 production during Lm infection

IL-12 serves as a cytokine critical for resistance to Lm infection, through its induction of IFN-γ (Tripp *et al.*, 1994). Several recent studies have questioned specifically whether DCs represent the source of Lm-induced IL-12 (Kapadia *et al.*, 2011; Mitchell *et al.*, 2011; Tam and Wick, 2006; Zhan *et al.*, 2010), and have generally agreed that both splenic CD8α^{+} DCs and monocyte-derived DCs serve are important producers of this cytokine. CD8α^{-} DCs have also been noted as a source of IL-12 in some of these reports. The microbial ligands generated by Lm that drive IL-12 production by these different cell types appear to be different, such that CD8α^{+} DCs seem to utilize redundant pathogen sensors that signal through MyD88, Trif, or Nod-like receptors (Zhan *et al.*, 2010). IL-12 production by monocyte-derived DCs, however, seems to critically depend on signals transmitted solely through MyD88. IL-12 drives clusters of NK cells within the white pulp to produce IFN-γ during the early phase of Lm infection, although this IFN-γ response also requires IL-18 (Kang *et al.*, 2008). The precise cellular source of IL-18 during *in vivo* Lm infection is unknown, although thioglycollate-elicited peritoneal macrophages produce this cytokine after Lm infection *in vitro* (Ozoren *et al.*, 2006). Interestingly, three manipulations result in both a lack of NK cell clustering and a failure of NK cells to produce IFN-γ (Kang *et al.*, 2008). DC deficiency blocks both of these NK cell responses, although the absence of PALS infection caused by this manipulation makes it difficult to assign DCs a specific role in mediating NK responses, given the larger role of DCs in Lm trafficking. MyD88 deficiency also blocks NK cell clustering and IFN-γ production, suggesting that numerous signals through MyD88, perhaps occurring in several cell types simultaneously, must all be working together to result in a full NK cell activation program. Third, cytosolic invasion by Lm is also required for NK cell clustering and IFN-γ production, suggesting a role for cytosolic sensors of Lm in this response.

4. DCS AS ANTIGEN-PRESENTING CELLS DURING LM INFECTION

Both CD4 and CD8 T cells can provide protective immunity to Lm infection, and so the question arises as to whether or not DCs are specifically involved as antigen-presenting cells (APCs), or whether other cell types serve as APCs to prime Lm-specific T cell responses. Given that LLO-secreting Lm can gain access to the host cell cytosol, presentation of Lm-derived peptides by MHC class I molecules could occur by infected cells via direct presentation. It is also possible, though, that exogenously derived Lm antigens might be cross-presented by uninfected DCs. Here, I will focus on a number of studies that have specifically examined the role of DCs in priming anti-Lm CD8 T cell responses. These priming events have been observed to occur within the white pulp of infected spleens (Aoshi *et al.*, 2008), the site of bacterial transport by $CD8\alpha^{+}$ DCs, as discussed above.

Given that systemic Lm infection results in bacterial replication within the cytosol of nonprofessional phagocytes (e.g., hepatocytes), an important observation came when it was determined that CD8 T cell priming to Lm required antigen presentation by a bone marrow-derived APC, rather than a parenchymal cell (Lenz *et al.*, 2000). Evidence for a specific role for DCs in this process was implied by the fact that mice treated with Flt3L to expand their DC populations *in vivo* primed a greater number of Lm-specific CD8 T cells (Alaniz *et al.*, 2004). This result, however, may have been due to the fact that these mice also had higher burdens of infection, and so potentially more antigen available for T cell priming.

Three studies examined CD8 T cell priming in DC-depleted CD11c-DTR transgenic mice. Two of these observed an absence of CD8 T cell priming when DCs were depleted before primary infection (Jung *et al.*, 2002; Muraille *et al.*, 2005), while one examined Lm-specific memory CD8 T cells and also saw markedly reduced proliferation of these cells during a secondary response to Lm (Zammit *et al.*, 2005). These studies failed to recognize, however, the profound resistance of DC-depleted mice to Lm infection (Neuenhahn *et al.*, 2006), which could have potentially explained these results as a reflection of decreased antigen load in DC-depleted mice, rather than a specific APC requirement. Importantly, upon infecting DC-depleted mice by way of injecting *ex vivo* Lm-infected bone marrow-derived macrophages, a manipulation shown to result in permissive *in vivo* infection in the absence of DCs, Neuenhahn *et al.* were able to effectively prime CD8 T cells to Lm. This result implies that APCs other than DCs can serve this function. Likewise, *Batf3*$^{-/-}$ mice fail to prime an Lm-specific CD8 T cell response at the typical inoculum used to infect wild-type mice, although these CD8α^+ DC-deficient mice do prime CD8 T cells effectively when higher inocula are used to adjust for equivalent bacterial burdens (Edelson *et al.*, 2011).

Nevertheless, a number of studies have shown CD8α^+ DCs to be particularly potent APCs during Lm infection (Campisi *et al.*, 2011; Lyszkiewicz *et al.*, 2011; Mitchell *et al.*, 2011). Mice deficient in the CD8α^+ DC-specific chemokine receptor Xcr1 display a defect in CD8 T cell priming, despite higher bacterial numbers in the spleen at day 3 after infection, also pointing to a role for CD8α^+ DCs in CD8 T cell priming (Crozat *et al.*, 2010). However, this study did not examine whether Lm transport to the PALS was normal in *Xcr1*$^{-/-}$ mice. Also relevant is a study examining CD8 T cell responses to Lm in transgenic mice expressing a mutant MHC class I molecule (H-2K^b) unable to traffic to endolysosomes, and therefore unable to acquire cross-presented antigen (Reinicke *et al.*, 2009). These mice showed lower, but not absent, levels of CD8 T cell priming after oral Lm infection, but their CD8 T cell responses were not examined after systemic infection. Results in *Batf3*$^{-/-}$ mice would imply that cross-presentation is not required to prime Lm-specific CD8 T cells, although cells other than CD8α^+ DCs can also efficiently present antigen on MHC class I via cross-presentation, particularly inflammatory monocytes (Segura *et al.*, 2009).

5. CONCLUSIONS

DCs play an important role during infection with many intracellular pathogens, including Lm. CD8α^+ DCs, in particular, play a unique role in this infection, serving as important hosts and transporters of the bacterium. Despite serving as an 'Achille's heel' in this system (Niedergang *et al.*, 2004), they also orchestrate a complicated interplay of other innate immune cells, including inflammatory monocytes and NK cells, and coordinate effective control of bacterial replication. Together with other APCs, they serve in the priming of T cell responses to Lm, which are necessary for sterilizing immunity. The study of DCs in Lm has revealed many nuances of their function that are applicable to understanding the biology of other infectious pathogens as well as to their potential function during vaccination. Undoubtedly, more DC mysteries in Lm infection are still to be revealed.

ACKNOWLEDGMENTS

I thank Tara Bradstreet, Javier Carrero, Emil Unanue, and Kenneth Murphy for many helpful discussions. My research is supported by a Burroughs Wellcome Fund Career Award for Medical Scientists and an American Society of Hematology Scholar Award.

NOTE ADDED IN PROOF

During the submission of this chapter, Verschoor *et al.* have reported that in the murine system, bloodborne Lm are rapidly opsonized by the complement factor C3, and subsequently associate with platelets via the platelet surface protein GPIb (Vershoor *et al.*, *Nat. Immunol.*, 2011 Oct 30. doi: 10.1038/ni.2140). This platelet association is required for efficient Lm infection of splenic CD8α+ DCs.

REFERENCES

Alaniz, R. C., Sandall, S., Thomas, E. K., and Wilson, C. B. (2004). Increased dendritic cell numbers impair protective immunity to intracellular bacteria despite augmenting antigen-specific CD8+ T lymphocyte responses. *J. Immunol.* **172,** 3725–3735.

Aoshi, T., Zinselmeyer, B. H., Konjufca, V., Lynch, J. N., Zhang, X., Koide, Y., and Miller, M. J. (2008). Bacterial entry to the splenic white pulp initiates antigen presentation to CD8+ T cells. *Immunity* **29,** 476–486.

Aoshi, T., Carrero, J. A., Konjufca, V., Koide, Y., Unanue, E. R., and Miller, M. J. (2009). The cellular niche of Listeria monocytogenes infection changes rapidly in the spleen. *Eur. J. Immunol.* **39,** 417–425.

Armstrong, B. A., and Sword, C. P. (1966). Electron microscopy of Listeria monocytogenes-infected mouse spleen. *J. Bacteriol.* **91,** 1346–1355.

Auerbuch, V., Brockstedt, D. G., Meyer-Morse, N., O'Riordan, M., and Portnoy, D. A. (2004). Mice lacking the type I interferon receptor are resistant to Listeria monocytogenes. *J. Exp. Med.* **200,** 527–533.

Bachem, A., Guttler, S., Hartung, E., Ebstein, F., Schaefer, M., Tannert, A., Salama, A., Movassaghi, K., Opitz, C., Mages, H. W., Henn, V., Kloetzel, P. M., *et al.* (2010). Superior antigen cross-presentation and XCR1 expression define human CD11c+CD141+ cells as homologues of mouse CD8+ dendritic cells. *J. Exp. Med.* **207,** 1273–1281.

Berche, P. (1995). Bacteremia is required for invasion of the murine central nervous system by Listeria monocytogenes. *Microb. Pathogen.* **18,** 323–336.

Bogunovic, M., Ginhoux, F., Helft, J., Shang, L., Hashimoto, D., Greter, M., Liu, K., Jakubzick, C., Ingersoll, M. A., Leboeuf, M., Stanley, E. R., Nussenzweig, M., *et al.* (2009). Origin of the lamina propria dendritic cell network. *Immunity* **31,** 513–525.

Campisi, L., Soudja, S. M., Cazareth, J., Bassand, D., Lazzari, A., Brau, F., Narni-Mancinelli, E., Glaichenhaus, N., Geissmann, F., and Lauvau, G. (2011). Splenic CD8alpha(+) dendritic cells undergo rapid programming by cytosolic bacteria and inflammation to induce protective CD8 memory. *Eur. J. Immunol.* **41,** 1594–1605.

Carrero, J. A., Calderon, B., and Unanue, E. R. (2004). Type I interferon sensitizes lymphocytes to apoptosis and reduces resistance to Listeria infection. *J. Exp. Med.* **200,** 535–540.

Chan, Y. Y., and Cheers, C. (1982). Mechanism of depletion of T lymphocytes from the spleen of mice infected with Listeria monocytogenes. *Infect. Immun.* **38,** 686–693.

Conlan, J. W. (1996). Early pathogenesis of Listeria monocytogenes infection in the mouse spleen. *J. Med. Microbiol.* **44,** 295–302.

Crozat, K., Guiton, R., Contreras, V., Feuillet, V., Dutertre, C. A., Ventre, E., Vu Manh, T. P., Baranek, T., Storset, A. K., Marvel, J., Boudinot, P., Hosmalin, A., *et al.* (2010). The XC chemokine receptor 1 is a conserved selective marker of mammalian cells homologous to mouse CD8alpha+ dendritic cells. *J. Exp. Med.* **207,** 1283–1292.

Disson, O., Grayo, S., Huillet, E., Nikitas, G., Langa-Vives, F., Dussurget, O., Ragon, M., Le Monnier, A., Babinet, C., Cossart, P., and Lecuit, M. (2008). Conjugated action of two species-specific invasion proteins for fetoplacental listeriosis. *Nature* **455,** 1114–1118.

Dresing, P., Borkens, S., Kocur, M., Kropp, S., and Scheu, S. (2010). A fluorescence reporter model defines "Tip-DCs" as the cellular source of interferon beta in murine listeriosis. *PLoS One* **5,** e15567.

Dudziak, D., Kamphorst, A. O., Heidkamp, G. F., Buchholz, V. R., Trumpfheller, C., Yamazaki, S., Cheong, C., Liu, K., Lee, H. W., Park, C. G., Steinman, R. M., and Nussenzweig, M. C. (2007). Differential antigen processing by dendritic cell subsets in vivo. *Science* **315,** 107–111.

Edelson, B. T., Kc, W., Juang, R., Kohyama, M., Benoit, L. A., Klekotka, P. A., Moon, C., Albring, J. C., Ise, W., Michael, D. G., Bhattacharya, D., Stappenbeck, T. S., *et al.* (2010). Peripheral CD103+ dendritic cells form a unified subset developmentally related to CD8alpha+ conventional dendritic cells. *J. Exp. Med.* **207,** 823–836.

Edelson, B. T., Bradstreet, T. R., Hildner, K., Carrero, J. A., Frederick, K. E., Kc, W., Belizaire, R., Aoshi, T., Schreiber, R. D., Miller, M. J., Murphy, T. L., Unanue, E. R., *et al.* (2011). CD8a+ dendritic cells are an obligate cellular entry point for productive infection by Listeria monocytogenes. *Immunity* **35,** 236–248.

Fogg, D. K., Sibon, C., Miled, C., Jung, S., Aucouturier, P., Littman, D. R., Cumano, A., and Geissmann, F. (2006). A clonogenic bone marrow progenitor specific for macrophages and dendritic cells. *Science* **311,** 83–87.

Geissmann, F., Gordon, S., Hume, D. A., Mowat, A. M., and Randolph, G. J. (2010a). Unravelling mononuclear phagocyte heterogeneity. *Nat. Rev. Immunol.* **10,** 453–460.

Geissmann, F., Manz, M. G., Jung, S., Sieweke, M. H., Merad, M., and Ley, K. (2010b). Development of monocytes, macrophages, and dendritic cells. *Science* **327,** 656–661.

Geurts van Kessel, C. H., Willart, M. A. M., van Rijt, L. S., Muskens, F., Kool, M., Baas, C., Thielemans, K., Bennett, C., Clasen, B. E., Hoogsteden, H. C., Osterhaus, A. D. M. E., Rimmelzwaan, G. F., *et al.* (2008). Clearance of influenza virus from the lung depends on migratory langerin(+)CD11b(−) but not plasmacytoid dendritic cells. *J. Exp. Med.* **205,** 1621–1634.

Ginhoux, F., Liu, K., Helft, J., Bogunovic, M., Greter, M., Hashimoto, D., Price, J., Yin, N., Bromberg, J., Lira, S. A., Stanley, E. R., Nussenzweig, M., *et al.* (2009). The origin and development of nonlymphoid tissue CD103+ DCs. *J. Exp. Med.* **206,** 3115–3130.

Gregory, S. H., Cousens, L. P., Van Rooijen, N., Dopp, E. A., Carlos, T. M., and Wing, E. J. (2002). Complementary adhesion molecules promote neutrophil-Kupffer cell interaction and the elimination of bacteria taken up by the liver. *J. Immunol.* **168,** 308–315.

Hardy, J., Francis, K. P., DeBoer, M., Chu, P., Gibbs, K., and Contag, C. H. (2004). Extracellular replication of Listeria monocytogenes in the murine gall bladder. *Science* **303,** 851–853.

Helft, J., Ginhoux, F., Bogunovic, M., and Merad, M. (2010). Origin and functional heterogeneity of non-lymphoid tissue dendritic cells in mice. *Immunol. Rev.* **234,** 55–75.

Hildner, K., Edelson, B. T., Purtha, W. E., Diamond, M., Matsushita, H., Kohyama, M., Calderon, B., Schraml, B. U., Unanue, E. R., Diamond, M. S., Schreiber, R. D., Murphy, T. L., *et al.* (2008). Batf3 deficiency reveals a critical role for CD8alpha+ dendritic cells in cytotoxic T cell immunity. *Science* **322,** 1097–1100.

Idoyaga, J., Suda, N., Suda, K., Park, C. G., and Steinman, R. M. (2009). Antibody to Langerin/CD207 localizes large numbers of CD8alpha+ dendritic cells to the marginal zone of mouse spleen. *Proc. Natl. Acad. Sci. USA* **106,** 1524–1529.

Jongbloed, S. L., Kassianos, A. J., McDonald, K. J., Clark, G. J., Ju, X. S., Angel, C. E., Chen, C. J. J., Dunbar, P. R., Wadley, R. B., Jeet, V., Vulink, A. J. E., Hart, D. N. J., *et al.* (2010). Human CD141(+) (BDCA-3)(+) dendritic cells (DCs) represent a unique myeloid DC subset that cross-presents necrotic cell antigens. *J. Exp. Med.* **207,** 1247–1260.

Jung, S., Unutmaz, D., Wong, P., Sano, G., De los, S. K., Sparwasser, T., Wu, S., Vuthoori, S., Ko, K., Zavala, F., Pamer, E. G., Littman, D. R., *et al.* (2002). In vivo depletion of CD11c(+) dendritic cells abrogates priming of CD8(+) T cells by exogenous cell-associated antigens. *Immunity* **17,** 211–220.

Kang, S. J., Liang, H. E., Reizis, B., and Locksley, R. M. (2008). Regulation of hierarchical clustering and activation of innate immune cells by dendritic cells. *Immunity* **29,** 819–833.

Kapadia, D., Sadikovic, A., Vanloubbeeck, Y., Brockstedt, D., and Fong, L. (2011). Interplay between CD8alpha dendritic cells and monocytes in response to Listeria monocytogenes infection attenuates T cell responses. *PLoS One* **6,** e19376.

Kraal, G., Breel, M., Janse, M., and Bruin, G. (1986). Langerhans cells, veiled cells, and interdigitating cells in the mouse recognized by a monoclonal antibody. *J. Exp. Med.* **163,** 981–997.

Lecuit, M., Vandormael-Pournin, S., Lefort, J., Huerre, M., Gounon, P., Dupuy, C., Babinet, C., and Cossart, P. (2001). A transgenic model for listeriosis: Role of internalin in crossing the intestinal barrier. *Science* **292,** 1722–1725.

Lenz, L. L., Butz, E. A., and Bevan, M. J. (2000). Requirements for bone marrow-derived antigen-presenting cells in priming cytotoxic T cell responses to intracellular pathogens. *J. Exp. Med.* **192,** 1135–1142.

Lin, M. L., Zhan, Y., Villadangos, J. A., and Lew, A. M. (2008). The cell biology of cross-presentation and the role of dendritic cell subsets. *Immunol. Cell Biol.* **86,** 353–362.

Liu, K., and Nussenzweig, M. C. (2010). Origin and development of dendritic cells. *Immunol. Rev.* **234,** 45–54.

Lyszkiewicz, M., Zietara, N., Rohde, M., Gekara, N. O., Jablonska, J., Dittmar, K. E., and Weiss, S. (2011). SIGN-R1+MHC II+ cells of the splenic marginal zone—A novel type of resident dendritic cells. *J. Leukoc. Biol.* **89,** 607–615.

Mebius, R. E., and Kraal, G. (2005). Structure and function of the spleen. *Nat. Rev. Immunol.* **5,** 606–616.

Merrick, J. C., Edelson, B. T., Bhardwaj, V., Swanson, P. E., and Unanue, E. R. (1997). Lymphocyte apoptosis during early phase of Listeria infection in mice. *Am. J. Pathol.* **151,** 785–792.

Mitchell, L. M., Brzoza-Lewis, K. L., Henry, C. J., Grayson, J. M., Westcott, M. M., and Hiltbold, E. M. (2011). Distinct responses of splenic dendritic cell subsets to infection

with Listeria monocytogenes: Maturation phenotype, level of infection, and T cell priming capacity ex vivo. *Cell. Immunol.* **268,** 79–86.
Muraille, E., Giannino, R., Guirnalda, P., Leiner, I., Jung, S., Pamer, E. G., and Lauvau, G. (2005). Distinct in vivo dendritic cell activation by live versus killed Listeria monocytogenes. *Eur. J. Immunol.* **35,** 1463–1471.
Muraille, E., Narni-Mancinelli, E., Gounon, P., Bassand, D., Glaichenhaus, N., Lenz, L. L., and Lauvau, G. (2007). Cytosolic expression of SecA2 is a prerequisite for long-term protective immunity. *Cell. Microbiol.* **9,** 1445–1454.
Naik, S. H., Sathe, P., Park, H. Y., Metcalf, D., Proietto, A. I., Dakic, A., Carotta, S., O'Keeffe, M., Bahlo, M., Papenfuss, A., Kwak, J. Y., Wu, L., *et al.* (2007). Development of plasmacytoid and conventional dendritic cell subtypes from single precursor cells derived in vitro and in vivo. *Nat. Immunol.* **8,** 1217–1226.
Neuenhahn, M., Kerksiek, K. M., Nauerth, M., Suhre, M. H., Schiemann, M., Gebhardt, F. E., Stemberger, C., Panthel, K., Schroder, S., Chakraborty, T., Jung, S., Hochrein, H., *et al.* (2006). CD8alpha+ dendritic cells are required for efficient entry of Listeria monocytogenes into the spleen. *Immunity* **25,** 619–630.
Niedergang, F., Didierlaurent, A., Kraehenbuhl, J. P., and Sirard, J. C. (2004). Dendritic cells: The host Achille's heel for mucosal pathogens? *Trends Microbiol.* **12,** 79–88.
O'Connell, R. M., Saha, S. K., Vaidya, S. A., Bruhn, K. W., Miranda, G. A., Zarnegar, B., Perry, A. K., Nguyen, B. O., Lane, T. F., Taniguchi, T., Miller, J. F., and Cheng, G. (2004). Type I interferon production enhances susceptibility to Listeria monocytogenes infection. *J. Exp. Med.* **200,** 437–445.
Onai, N., Obata-Onai, A., Schmid, M. A., Ohteki, T., Jarrossay, D., and Manz, M. G. (2007). Identification of clonogenic common Flt3(+) M-CSFR+ plasmacytoid and conventional dendritic cell progenitors in mouse bone marrow. *Nat. Immunol.* **8,** 1207–1216.
Ozoren, N., Masumoto, J., Franchi, L., Kanneganti, T. D., Body-Malapel, M., Erturk, I., Jagirdar, R., Zhu, L., Inohara, N., Bertin, J., Coyle, A., Grant, E. P., *et al.* (2006). Distinct roles of TLR2 and the adaptor ASC in IL-1beta/IL-18 secretion in response to Listeria monocytogenes. *J. Immunol.* **176,** 4337–4342.
Poulin, L. F., Salio, M., Griessinger, E., Anjos-Afonso, F., Craciun, L., Chen, J. L., Keller, A. M., Joffre, O., Zelenay, S., Nye, E., Le Moine, A., Faure, F., *et al.* (2010). Characterization of human DNGR-1+ BDCA3+ leukocytes as putative equivalents of mouse CD8alpha+ dendritic cells. *J. Exp. Med.* **207,** 1261–1271.
Pron, B., Boumaila, C., Jaubert, F., Berche, P., Milon, G., Geissmann, F., and Gaillard, J. L. (2001). Dendritic cells are early cellular targets of Listeria monocytogenes after intestinal delivery and are involved in bacterial spread in the host. *Cell. Microbiol.* **3,** 331–340.
Reinicke, A. T., Omilusik, K. D., Basha, G., and Jefferies, W. A. (2009). Dendritic cell cross-priming is essential for immune responses to Listeria monocytogenes. *PLoS One* **4,** e7210.
Sathaliyawala, T., O'Gorman, W. E., Greter, M., Bogunovic, M., Konjufca, V., Hou, Z. E., Nolan, G. P., Miller, M. J., Merad, M., and Reizis, B. (2010). Mammalian target of rapamycin controls dendritic cell development downstream of Flt3 ligand signaling. *Immunity* **33,** 597–606.
Segura, E., Albiston, A. L., Wicks, I. P., Chai, S. Y., and Villadangos, J. A. (2009). Different cross-presentation pathways in steady-state and inflammatory dendritic cells. *Proc. Natl. Acad. Sci. USA* **106,** 20377–20381.
Serbina, N. V., Salazar-Mather, T. P., Biron, C. A., Kuziel, W. A., and Pamer, E. G. (2003). TNF/iNOS-producing dendritic cells mediate innate immune defense against bacterial infection. *Immunity* **19,** 59–70.
Serbina, N. V., Jia, T., Hohl, T. M., and Pamere, E. G. (2008). Monocyte-mediated defense against microbial pathogens. *Annu. Rev. Immunol.* **26,** 421–452.

Solodova, E., Jablonska, J., Weiss, S., and Lienenklaus, S. (2011). Production of IFN-beta during Listeria monocytogenes infection is restricted to monocyte/macrophage lineage. *PLoS One* **6,** e18543.

Stavru, F., Archambaud, C., and Cossart, P. (2011). Cell biology and immunology of Listeria monocytogenes infections: Novel insights. *Immunol. Rev.* **240,** 160–184.

Stockinger, S., Kastner, R., Kernbauer, E., Pilz, A., Westermayer, S., Reutterer, B., Soulat, D., Stengl, G., Vogl, C., Frenz, T., Waibler, Z., Taniguchi, T., *et al.* (2009). Characterization of the interferon-producing cell in mice infected with Listeria monocytogenes. *PLoS Pathog.* **5,** e1000355.

Swiecki, M., and Colonna, M. (2010). Unraveling the functions of plasmacytoid dendritic cells during viral infections, autoimmunity, and tolerance. *Immunol. Rev.* **234,** 142–162.

Tam, M. A., and Wick, M. J. (2006). Differential expansion, activation and effector functions of conventional and plasmacytoid dendritic cells in mouse tissues transiently infected with Listeria monocytogenes. *Cell. Microbiol.* **8,** 1172–1187.

Tripp, C. S., Gately, M. K., Hakimi, J., Ling, P., and Unanue, E. R. (1994). Neutralization of IL-12 decreases resistance to Listeria in SCID and C.B-17 mice. Reversal by IFN-gamma. *J. Immunol.* **152,** 1883–1887.

Wollert, T., Pasche, B., Rochon, M., Deppenmeier, S., van den, H. J., Gruber, A. D., Heinz, D. W., Lengeling, A., and Schubert, W. D. (2007). Extending the host range of Listeria monocytogenes by rational protein design. *Cell* **129,** 891–902.

Xu, Y., Zhan, Y., Lew, A. M., Naik, S. H., and Kershaw, M. H. (2007). Differential development of murine dendritic cells by GM-CSF versus Flt3 ligand has implications for inflammation and trafficking. *J. Immunol.* **179,** 7577–7584.

Zammit, D. J., Cauley, L. S., Pham, Q. M., and Lefrancois, L. (2005). Dendritic cells maximize the memory CD8 T cell response to infection. *Immunity* **22,** 561–570.

Zhan, Y., Xu, Y., Seah, S., Brady, J. L., Carrington, E. M., Cheers, C., Croker, B. A., Wu, L., Villadangos, J. A., and Lew, A. M. (2010). Resident and monocyte-derived dendritic cells become dominant IL-12 producers under different conditions and signaling pathways. *J. Immunol.* **185,** 2125–2133.

Zhan, Y., Carrington, E. M., van Nieuwenhuijze, A., Bedoui, S., Seah, S., Xu, Y., Wang, N., Mintern, J. D., Villadangos, J. A., Wicks, I. P., and Lew, A. M. (2011). GM-CSF increases cross presentation and CD103 expression by mouse CD8(+) spleen dendritic cells. *Eur. J. Immunol.* **41,** 2585–2595.

CHAPTER 5

Probing CD8 T Cell Responses with *Listeria monocytogenes* Infection

Stephanie A. Condotta,[*,1] **Martin J. Richer,**[†,1] **Vladimir P. Badovinac,**[*,‡,1] and **John T. Harty**[*,†,‡,1]

Contents

* Department of Pathology, University of Iowa, Iowa City, Iowa, USA
† Department of Microbiology, University of Iowa, Iowa City, Iowa, USA
‡ Interdisciplinary Graduate Program in Immunology, University of Iowa, Iowa City, Iowa, USA
[1] Authors contributed equally.

Advances in Immunology, Volume 113
ISSN 0065-2776, DOI: 10.1016/B978-0-12-394590-7.00005-1

Abstract

CD8 T cells play a critical role in the control and eradication of intracellular pathogens. Increased understanding of CD8 T cell biology provides insight that can be translated into improved vaccination strategies. The intracellular bacterium, *Listeria monocytogenes*, has been used as a model organism to study every phase of the CD8 T cell response to intracellular bacterial infection. Infection of laboratory mice with *L. monocytogenes* has provided insight into the factors that are involved in primary T cell responses, memory CD8 T cell generation, maintenance, functionality, and diversification following repeated pathogenic challenges. In this review, we will focus on work from our laboratories utilizing the murine model of *L. monocytogenes* to investigate the characteristics of CD8 T cell responses to infection. This model has profoundly advanced our understanding of the CD8 T cell response to infection and is likely to continue to provide invaluable basic insights that can be translated into the development of effective vaccination strategies to protect against pathogens.

1. INTRODUCTION

Listeria monocytogenes, first described in 1926 (Murray *et al.*, 1926), is a Gram-positive food-borne pathogen that is the etiological agent of listeriosis. Listeriosis results in diverse clinical manifestations, which can be attributed to the capacity of *L. monocytogenes* to cross three tight barriers within the human host (Stavru *et al.*, 2011; Wing and Gregory, 2000). Following the ingestion of contaminated food, *L. monocytogenes* is able to cross the intestinal barrier and invade the intestinal epithelium, resulting in gastroenteritis. In addition, *L. monocytogenes* has the unique ability to cross the feto-placental barrier in pregnant women. This can lead to infection of the fetus and septic abortion. Finally, *L. monocytogenes* has the capability to cross the blood–brain barrier and infect the meninges in the brain, resulting in potentially fatal meningitis and encephalitis (Pamer, 2004).

Due to its capacity to trigger uptake into cells that normally lack phagocytic capacities, this remarkable bacterium is able to infect a large variety of cell types (Hamon *et al.*, 2006). Once inside the host cell, *L. monocytogenes* escapes the phagosome by secreting the pore forming toxin listeriolysin O (LLO), thus gaining access to the host cell cytosol. Within the cytosol, bacterial replication begins and the recruitment and polymerization of cellular actin are induced. Mobility within the cytosol is mediated by polar expression of the bacterial nucleating actin protein, actin-assembly-inducing protein (ActA). This provides *L. monocytogenes* a scaffold of polymerized F-actin to propel itself through the cytoplasm, ultimately reaching the plasma membrane. As a consequence, long protrusions containing bacteria are created and these can be invaginated by neighboring cells, enabling *L. monocytogenes* to continue its replication process within a newly infected cell. *L. monocytogenes* strains that have been genetically manipulated to delete the *actA* gene have drastically reduced pathogenicity *in vivo*. Importantly, this mode of direct cell-to-cell spread allows *L. monocytogenes* to largely avoid the extracellular milieu thereby escaping the neutralizing effects of antibodies and of the complement system (Hamon *et al.*, 2006). Although *L. monocytogenes* has evolved clever ways to manipulate the host cell to its advantage, its presence within the host cell cytosol can be recognized by the immune system and induces a potent CD8 T cell response (Harty and Bevan, 1999; Lara-Tejero and Pamer, 2004). This response ultimately results in clearance of the bacterial infection and subsequent acquisition of life-long protective immunity.

L. monocytogenes infection in animal models has been a useful tool to evaluate host–pathogen interactions. Intravenous inoculation of *L. monocytogenes* into laboratory mice has been utilized as a model system for decades to investigate intracellular bacterial infections. In pioneering studies at the Trudeau Institute in the 1960s, Mackaness and coworkers used *L. monocytogenes* infection to demonstrate the central role of cellular immunity in controlling infection with an intracellular pathogen (Mackaness, 1962, 1964). This seminal work paved the way for many important immunological discoveries using the murine model of listeriosis. As will be discussed below, these studies have led to the development of murine listeriosis as perhaps the most utilized animal model to investigate host defense against intracellular bacterial pathogens. Using this model, multiple research groups have made important observations to further our understanding of CD8 T cell biology. This review will focus primarily on the work from our laboratories utilizing the murine model of listeriosis to evoke and study all facets of the CD8 T cell responses to intracellular bacterial infection.

2. RECOMBINANT *L. MONOCYTOGENES* AS A VERSATILE VEHICLE TO PROBE ANTIGEN-SPECIFIC CD8 T CELL RESPONSES

The murine model of *L. monocytogenes* infection represents a unique tool that has advanced our knowledge of all aspects of CD8 T cell responses to infection with intracellular pathogens. Specifically, the *L. monocytogenes* murine model has at least three major strengths that, as described below, have allowed for several key findings into the biology of CD8 T cell responses to infection.

First, the bacterium has been successfully engineered to express model antigens, thus expanding the "toolkit" for immunological studies. Second, the generation of *L. monocytogenes* with attenuated pathogenicity has allowed for the use of this bacterium to elicit CD8 T cell responses in immunocompromised mice that would otherwise be highly susceptible to infection. Third, the capacity to manipulate the duration of *L. monocytogenes* infection with antibiotics has facilitated studies regarding the role of inflammation and antigen presentation for both expansion and contraction of CD8 T cells. These advantages have made *L. monocytogenes* one of the most versatile and widely used pathogens to elicit and study essentially all phases of CD8 T cell responses to infection.

Early studies of CD8 T cell responses to infection were hampered by a lack of knowledge of specific CD8 T cell epitopes. This situation was partially rectified with the identification of epitopes from the LLO (Pamer *et al.*, 1991) and p60 (Pamer, 1994) antigens recognized by CD8 T cells in BALB/c mice. This is one specific area where the versatility of the *L. monocytogenes* murine model has allowed major advances. Pioneering studies involving our groups and others have demonstrated that *L. monocytogenes* could be engineered to express known CD8 T cell epitopes from other pathogens or model antigens (Schafer *et al.*, 1992; Shen *et al.*, 1995, 1998). For example, *L. monocytogenes* was engineered to express a lymphocytic choriomeningitis virus (LCMV) nucleoprotein epitope ($NP_{118-126}$) in either a secreted or a nonsecreted form. Interestingly, both versions of this epitope were able to prime a CD8 T cell response (Shen *et al.*, 1998). This was surprising, as epitopes from nonsecreted *L. monocytogenes* antigens had not been reported, suggesting that only secreted antigens were able to prime CD8 T cell responses. Importantly, while NP_{118}-specific CD8 T cells primed by LCMV infection protected against *L. monocytogenes* expressing the secreted viral antigen, they were unable to protect from infection with an *L. monocytogenes* strain expressing the nonsecreted form of the antigen. This demonstrated an important dichotomy between the capacity of a specific antigen to prime CD8 T cells and the ability of that antigen to serve as a target for protective CD8 T cell responses. Specifically, this study revealed that antigenic compartmentalization in bacteria is a fundamental consideration for the selection of protective antigens. In addition, this study highlights the usefulness of *L. monocytogenes* strains, genetically manipulated to express heterologous antigen, to probe antigen-specific CD8 T cell responses.

Subsequently, *L. monocytogenes* has been engineered to express a well-defined ovalbumin (OVA) epitope (LM-OVA) that permits studies in C57BL/6 mice and the application of the OVA-specific T cell receptor (TCR) transgenic T cell (OT-I) (Hogquist *et al.*, 1994; Pope *et al.*, 2001). Additionally, recombinant *L. monocytogenes* strains expressing LCMV glycoprotein (GP_{33-41}) (Kaech and Ahmed, 2001; San Mateo *et al.*, 2002), *Plasmodium yoelii* circumsporozoite ($CS_{280-288}$) (Schmidt *et al.*, 2008), and influenza A hemagglutinin ($HA_{518-526}$) (Pham *et al.*, 2010) have been engineered to facilitate studies with P14 (Pircher *et al.*, 1987), CS TCR transgenic (Sano *et al.*, 2001), and Clone 4 TCR transgenic T cells (Morgan *et al.*, 1996). As discussed below, this system has been used in several studies to advance our knowledge of CD8 T cell responses.

Another major contribution of the *L. monocytogenes* murine model has been the application of genetically attenuated strains to probe the importance of several immune genes for CD8 T cell responses to infection. The majority of pathogens including wild-type *L. monocytogenes* cannot be used to probe CD8 T cell responses in knockout (KO) mice lacking specific immune genes, as these mouse strains are highly susceptible to infection. For example, we showed that interferon-gamma (IFN-γ)-deficient mice, on the BALB/c background, are highly susceptible to infection with wild-type *L. monocytogenes* ($LD_{50} < 10$ bacteria). However, IFN-γ-deficient mice were able to survive and clear infection with an attenuated strain of *L. monocytogenes* lacking the *actA* gene (DPL1942, $LD_{50} > 1{,}000{,}000$ bacteria) (Harty and Bevan, 1995). We used this approach to show that, in contrast to the previous literature (Buchmeier and Schreiber, 1985; Huang *et al.*, 1993), CD8 T cells lacking the capacity to produce IFN-γ could still protect mice from reinfection with wild-type *L. monocytogenes*. Perhaps more importantly, this study demonstrated that attenuated strains of *L. monocytogenes* could be used to probe CD8 T cell responses in mice lacking specific immune genes thereby opening a previously untapped resource. As described below, the use of attenuated strains of *L. monocytogenes* to infect mice deficient for specific immune genes has played an integral role in major discoveries at all phases of CD8 T cell responses to infection.

Another important advantage of the *L. monocytogenes* model is the capacity to modulate the duration of infection. As opposed to viral pathogens that have been used to probe CD8 T cell responses, *L. monocytogenes* infection can be rapidly terminated through the use of antibiotic treatment. In addition, studies from our group and others have demonstrated that pretreatment of mice with antibiotic yields a very short course of infection with substantially reduced levels of inflammation (Badovinac *et al.*, 2002, 2004; Mercado *et al.*, 2000). This approach has been used to answer fundamental question relating the role of both duration of infection and inflammation in the expansion, contraction, and transition to memory of antigen-specific CD8 T cells. These advantages have made *L. monocytogenes* murine model a workhorse for studies aimed at understanding CD8 T cell responses to infection. As detailed below, the unique advantages of this system have been exploited to increase our understanding of all phases of CD8 T cells responding to infection.

3. PRIMARY CD8 T CELL RESPONSES

3.1. CD8 T cell expansion

3.1.1. Programming of T cell expansion

The naive repertoire of CD8 T cells specific for a particular antigen constitutes but a very small fraction of the total CD8 compartment, ranging from approximately 10 to 1000 cells in an inbred laboratory mouse (Blattman *et al.*, 2002; Casrouge *et al.*, 2000; Moon *et al.*, 2007; Obar *et al.*, 2008). As such, CD8 T cells must undergo a massive numerical expansion in order to properly defend against infection with rapidly proliferating pathogens. Following recognition of cognate antigen presented by mature dendritic cells (DCs), CD8 T cell numbers can expand >10,000-fold (Fig. 5.1) (Badovinac and Harty, 2002; Butz and Bevan, 1998; Murali-Krishna *et al.*, 1998). Classically, CD8 T cell expansion was believed to correlate with antigen persistence and to be maintained until T cells somehow sensed the disappearance of antigen. However, experiments taking advantage of the capacity to modulate the duration of *L. monocytogenes* infection have challenged this notion.

Experiments by Mercado *et al.* demonstrated that the expansion phase of the CD8 T cell response was largely unaffected in mice where *L. monocytogenes* infection was prematurely truncated by antibiotic treatment starting at 24 h postinfection (Mercado *et al.*, 2000). Interestingly, the expansion of CD8 T cells was significantly reduced when antibiotic treatment was started 12 h after infection (Mercado *et al.*, 2000). These experiments strongly suggested that, following a set but short window of stimulation, continued expansion of CD8 T cells is not dependent on the presence of infectious agent or antigen. Rather, these cells are rapidly programmed to undergo many rounds of division following an initial period of stimulation. These results were confirmed by studies in our laboratories (Badovinac *et al.*, 2002) and extended to demonstrate that expansion of CD4 T cells was similarly programmed during the early stages of infections (Corbin and Harty, 2004). In strong support of these observations, several groups have demonstrated *in vitro* that the capacity to undergo several rounds of division and to acquire effector functions can be programmed following as little as 2 h of antigenic stimulation (Kaech and Ahmed, 2001; van Stipdonk *et al.*, 2001; Wong and Pamer, 2001). Taken together, these data demonstrated that, while later events are likely to exert an influence on responding antigen-specific T cells (Bevan, 2004; Sun *et al.*, 2004), a short period of antigen stimulation is sufficient to activate a program of T cell expansion that continues for multiple rounds of cell division independently of further antigenic stimulation.

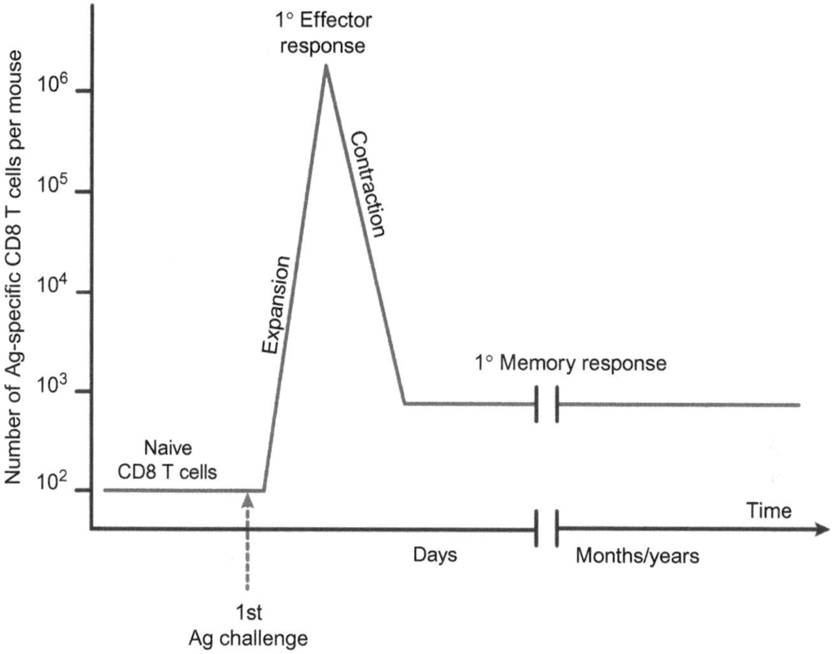

FIGURE 5.1 Kinetics of CD8 T cell responses to *L. monocytogenes* infection. Upon recognition of their cognate antigen presented by a mature DC, antigen-specific naive CD8 T cells undergo massive numerical proliferation (expansion), whereby the T cell numbers expand >10,000-fold. Subsequently, the CD8 T cells acquire effector functions (1° effector response) such as cytolytic activity and the capability to produce cytokines. Following the peak of expansion, the antigen-experienced effector CD8 T cells rapidly contract in numbers, resulting in death of 90–95% of the responding T cells (Contraction). The 5–10% of cells that survive the initial contraction phase constitute the primary memory CD8 T cell pool (1° memory response). The remaining antigen-specific memory CD8 T cells provide life-long protective immunity from reinfection (Ag, antigen). (For color version of this figure, the reader is referred to the Web version of this chapter.)

3.1.2. Effector molecules and CD8 T cell expansion

Following antigen stimulation, CD8 T cells acquire the capacity to exert effector functions through the expression of molecules such as granzyme B and perforin and the capacity to produce cytokines such as IFN-γ and tumor necrosis factor-alpha (TNF-α) (Harty and Badovinac, 2002). While the role of these molecules in the clearance of invading pathogens is clearly established (Bancroft *et al.*, 1989; Buchmeier and Schreiber, 1985; Harty *et al.*, 2000; Huang *et al.*, 1993; Rothe *et al.*, 1993), several lines of evidence also point to a role for these effector molecules in CD8 T cell homeostasis over the course of infection. Taking advantage of the reduced pathogenicity of attenuated *L. monocytogenes* even in mice lacking specific immune genes (Harty and Bevan, 1995), studies from our laboratories have demonstrated that perforin deficiency yields a three- to fourfold increase in the expansion of CD8 T cells specific for two *L. monocytogenes* epitopes ($LLO_{91–99}$ and $p60_{217–225}$) (Badovinac *et al.*, 2000). The attenuated strain of *L. monocytogenes* (*actA* deficient) used in this study was cleared with similar kinetics in perforin-deficient and wild-type mice, suggesting that the increase in expansion was independent of an increase in the duration of infection. This demonstrated that perforin plays an important role in regulating T cell expansion independently of its role in bacterial clearance. Similar increases in T cell expansion were also observed in models of viral infection, such as LCMV, in perforin KO mice (Kagi *et al.*, 1999; Matloubian *et al.*, 1999).

Together these studies demonstrated that in addition to playing an important role in bacterial clearance, the capacity of T cell to produce perforin represents a regulatory mechanism that might be important to prevent overexpansion of antigen-specific CD8 T cells. The underlying molecular mechanisms determining the role of perforin in CD8 T cells homeostasis remain poorly defined but may be related to the leakage of granular content such as granzyme B leading to the death of activated T cells. In support of this notion, mice expressing increased levels of the granzyme B inhibitor, serine protease inhibitor 6, have a similar increased T cell expansion following LCMV infection (Phillips *et al.*, 2004). This suggests that perforin expression by CD8 T cells may represent an autocrine regulatory mechanism that may be critical to prevent immunopathology and/or the induction of autoimmunity following infection.

Absence of the critical effector cytokine IFN-γ has also been demonstrated to regulate CD8 T cell expansion following *L. monocytogenes* infection. Interestingly, the expansion of CD8 T cells specific for the immunodominant epitope $LLO_{91–99}$ and for CD8 T cells specific for the subdominant epitope $p60_{217–225}$, as measured using specific $H2\text{-}K^d$ tetramers (Busch *et al.*, 1998), was affected differently in IFN-γ-deficient mice (Badovinac *et al.*, 2000). This resulted in an overall shift in the usually strictly conserved immunodominance hierarchy. Immunodominance is generally believed to relate to the frequency of naive T cell precursors, strength of TCR and major histocompatibility complex (MHC) interactions, and antigen availability (Yewdell and Bennink, 1999). However, these three components are unlikely to be affected by the deficiency of IFN-γ. On the other hand, IFN-γ has also been demonstrated to play a role in the expression of several proteasome subunits, and as such, absence of IFN-γ is likely to impact protein degradation and the generation of specific epitopes, potentially explaining how this effector cytokine can regulate immunodominance (Fruh and Yang, 1999). Consistent with the idea, it was shown that the absence of IFN-γ influences the relative prevalence of antigenic peptides derived from *L. monocytogenes in vivo* (Skoberne and Geginat, 2002). Taken together, these data demonstrate that the effector functions of CD8 T cell can also play an integral role in regulation of CD8 T cell expansion in response to infection. It will remain of interest to determine whether other effector functions of CD8 T cells are also involved in autocrine regulatory loops affecting overall CD8 T cell expansion.

3.1.3. Inflammation and CD8 T cell expansion

The cytokine milieu at the time of T cell activation also plays an important role in the expansion phase of the CD8 T cell response. In addition to signals 1 and 2 provided by DCs, CD8 T cells also require a third signal in order to achieve optimal accumulation (Curtsinger and Mescher, 2010). Several studies have demonstrated that systemic inflammation provides this third signal directly to responding T cells (Aichele *et al.*, 2006; Curtsinger *et al.*, 2003; Havenar-Daughton *et al.*, 2006; Kolumam *et al.*, 2005; Whitmire *et al.*, 2005). Pretreatment with antibiotics dramatically reduced the levels of inflammatory cytokines induced following *L. monocytogenes* infection and resulted in a lower number of antigen-specific CD8 T cells at the peak of the response (Badovinac *et al.*, 2004). Further evidence has demonstrated that T cells lacking the capacity to respond to interleukin 12 (IL-12) are also impaired during the expansion phase of the response following *L. monocytogenes* infection (Pearce and Shen, 2007), while in the case of other infections such as LCMV, accumulation is mostly regulated by the presence of type I interferons (Aichele *et al.*, 2006; Kolumam *et al.*, 2005).

Taken together, these data highlight the importance of signal 3 cytokines for the accumulation of antigen-specific CD8 T cells following infection with various pathogens. Interestingly, these studies also demonstrated that multiple cytokines can serve as signal 3 depending on the invading pathogen (Thompson *et al.*, 2006). The mechanism explaining how signal 3 cytokines lead to optimal accumulation of responding T cells remains to be fully understood. *In vitro* studies have suggested that both IL-12 and type I interferons can enhance survival of T cells (Curtsinger *et al.*, 1999; Marrack *et al.*, 1999; Xiao *et al.*, 2009). While these data suggest that, in some systems, signal 3 cytokines may serve to enhance T cell survival, it will remain important to further investigate the effects of signal 3 cytokines on both the accumulation and the overall function of responding T cells. Recent evidence from our laboratory has demonstrated that signal 3 cytokines are also important for optimal accumulation of CD8 T cells following DC immunization (Pham *et al.*, 2011). This minimalist system will likely prove invaluable to further dissect the role of various inflammatory stimuli in CD8 T cell responses.

3.2. CD8 T cell contraction

3.2.1. Programming of CD8 T cell contraction

Following peak expansion, CD8 T cells undergo a rapid transition to a contraction phase that results in the death of 90–95% of the effector population. As the cells that survive contraction will go on to establish a memory population (Fig. 5.1), understanding the factors that dictate the survival of certain cells during this phase of the response has important implications for the design of effective vaccines. Following infection with various pathogens, the onset of contraction was observed to correlate with pathogen clearance. This was initially interpreted as responding T cells somehow sensing the disappearance of antigen and responding by initiating a program ultimately resulting in cell death. However, in certain infection models, such as chronic viral infections, pathogen persistence did not abrogate contraction (Badovinac *et al.*, 2002; Fuller *et al.*, 2004; Wherry *et al.*, 2004). This suggested that T cell contraction is not regulated by pathogen persistence.

To address the link between length of infection and the onset of contraction, we infected mice with *L. monocytogenes* and terminated the infection with antibiotic treatment (Badovinac *et al.*, 2002, 2004). Early termination of *L. monocytogenes* infection with antibiotic at 24 h postinfection was not sufficient to change the kinetics or magnitude of the contraction phase (Badovinac *et al.*, 2002). This clearly demonstrated that clearance of infection and the onset of contraction are not directly linked and that even a shortened period of antigenic interaction is sufficient to program responding T cells to undergo contraction. Further experiments in the murine model of listeriosis have demonstrated that inflammation plays a critical role in programming contraction of T cells. Pretreatment of mice with antibiotics significantly reduces the level of inflammatory cytokines, including IFN-γ, induced following *L. monocytogenes* infection. This resulted in a substantial reduction in the contraction phase of the CD8 T cell response (Badovinac *et al.*, 2004). Interestingly, while deficiency of IFN-γ resulted in relatively normal expansion of CD8 T cells following *actA*-deficient *L. monocytogenes* infection, contraction was severely abrogated (Badovinac *et al.*, 2000). In support of this notion, induction of inflammatory cytokines with Toll-like receptor (TLR) agonist such as CpG is sufficient to increase contraction in mice which had been pretreated with antibiotics (Badovinac *et al.*, 2004).

Interestingly, manipulation of the duration of infection with either attenuated or virulent (wild type) strains of *L. monocytogenes* has demonstrated that contraction is usually programmed to initiate approximately 5 days following the peak of "functional" antigen presentation further supporting the idea that contraction is programmed early during antigenic stimulation (Porter and Harty, 2006). These data demonstrate an important role for inflammatory cytokines in the induction of a program ultimately resulting in the contraction of responding CD8 T cells although the exact mechanisms through which cytokines such as IFN-γ can regulate contraction remain to be fully elucidated. The mechanism may in part relate to the induction of the expression of molecules such as the proapoptotic molecule Bim (Pellegrini *et al.*, 2003; Prlic and Bevan, 2008). As such, contraction appears to be programmed early after antigenic encounter and is largely controlled by the induction of systemic inflammation.

3.2.2. Factors determining survival from contraction

Another important consideration that has been the subject of intense investigation relates to the identification of the factors allowing some CD8 T cells to survive the contraction phase and go on to establish memory. One long debated hypothesis centers on the competition for important survival factors such as the cytokine IL-7. Interestingly, while the majority of antigen-specific T cells downregulate the expression of the IL-7 receptor α chain (IL-7Rα) during the expansion phase, a small number of cells maintain the expression of IL-7Rα (Kaech *et al.*, 2003). Importantly, this population correlates with the number of cells surviving to the memory phase suggesting that IL-7Rα expression identifies CD8 T cells with the potential to become memory cells. Further, this strongly suggested that IL-7 mediated survival signals may be involved in allowing cells to survive contraction and become long-lived memory cells. However, we have demonstrated that constitutive expression of IL-7Rα by CD8 T cells is not sufficient to prevent contraction of T cells following *L. monocytogenes* infection (Haring *et al.*, 2008). Similar results were observed in an LCMV infection model (Hand *et al.*, 2007) and increased IL-7 signaling was not sufficient to increase memory formation following LCMV infection (Sun *et al.*, 2006).

Additionally, induction of CD8 T cell responses under conditions leading to low systemic inflammation such as DC immunization or peptide vaccination results in a much greater proportion of T cells maintaining expression of IL-7Rα while contraction is minimally affected (Badovinac *et al.*, 2005; Lacombe *et al.*, 2005; Pham *et al.*, 2009, 2010). Thus, competition for IL-7 is not sufficient to explain the induction of the contraction phase. This suggests that while cells that survive into the memory phase may maintain expression IL-7Rα throughout the course of the response, expression of this cytokine receptor is not sufficient to enforce survival during the contraction phase. Further experiments will be required in order to better understand the mechanistic events that lead to certain T cells surviving the contraction phase. Understanding the factors that lead to a highly reproducible fraction of CD8 T cells surviving contraction and establishing memory populations is likely to be of critical importance for the optimization of vaccines that generate optimal memory populations.

4. MEMORY CD8 T CELL RESPONSES

Immunological memory is a hallmark of the adaptive immune system and a primary goal of vaccine development. Therefore, increased understanding of all aspects of memory generation and maintenance is critical for the development of effective vaccination strategies. The basis of vaccination is built upon the ability of the immune system to mount a robust and rapid recall response following subsequent exposure to a pathogen (Nolz and Harty, 2012). Life-long protective immunity is dependent upon the quantity and quality of the memory T cell pool (Harty and Badovinac, 2008; Kaech *et al.*, 2002a; Schmidt *et al.*, 2008, 2010). The CD8 T cells that survive following contraction initiate the memory pool and these cells have unique features allowing them to survive long term and provide protection from reinfection. Understanding the factors that influence memory CD8 T cell generation, homeostasis, and functionality has been a focus in our laboratories for many years. The many advantages of the *L. monocytogenes* murine model have allowed our groups and others to probe the requirements for the generation, maintenance, and functionality of both primary and multiply stimulated memory CD8 T cells. Some of the major insights stemming from the *L. monocytogenes* murine model will be discussed in the following sections.

4.1. Memory CD8 T cell generation

As described above, 5–10% of antigen-experienced effector CD8 T cells survive contraction and constitute the initial memory CD8 T cell pool (Fig. 5.1) (Badovinac and Harty, 2006). While there is no single phenotypic marker that defines memory T cells, methods have been developed to help characterize the changing phenotype of CD8 T cells that progresses from naive ($CD62L^{hi}$, $CCR7^{hi}$, IL-7Rα^{hi}, IFN-γ^{low}, and IL-2^{low}) to effector ($CD62L^{low}$, $CCR7^{low}$, IL-7Rα^{low}, and IFN-γ^{hi}, IL-2^{low}) to memory ($CD62L^{low/hi}$, $CCR7^{low/hi}$, IL-7Rα^{hi}, IFN-γ^{hi}, and IL-$2^{low/hi}$) (Badovinac and Harty, 2006). Importantly, substantial heterogeneity exists even within a population of memory CD8 T cells specific for a single epitope (Jameson and Masopust, 2009). The memory CD8 T cell pool can be grossly separated into two populations based on the expression levels of the lymph node homing markers CD62L and CCR7. This has led to memory populations being divided into effector memory (T_{EM}) ($CD62L^{low}$ and $CCR7^{low}$) and central memory (T_{CM}) ($CD62L^{hi}$ and $CCR7^{hi}$) subsets (Sallusto *et al.*, 1999; Wherry *et al.*, 2003). Expression of CD62L and CCR7 drastically changes the homing characteristics of these two populations with T_{EM} predominately localizing within peripheral tissues while T_{CM} retain the capacity to home to lymphoid organs (Masopust *et al.*, 2001). Upon antigen reencounter, both subsets are able to rapidly produce cytokines such as IFN-γ and TNF-α while responding T_{CM} also produce IL-2 (Wherry *et al.*, 2003). Additionally, although both subsets are able to proliferate in response to antigen reencounter, T_{CM} are generally observed to expand more vigorously than T_{EM} (Wherry *et al.*, 2003). Ideally, an effective memory T cell population should persist in higher numbers than the naive population, respond and expand rapidly, and provide enhanced protection to pathogen reencounter.

Understanding the mechanistic requirements for the development of effective CD8 memory T cells may provide important insights into how this process can be manipulated in order to generate highly protective vaccine strategies. Understanding how to enhance or expedite the rate of memory formation would likely result in the generation of more effective vaccine approaches. The rate of memory progression is not static and is pathogen dependent. For example, conversion to a T_{CM} phenotype occurs relatively rapidly (1–2 months) following infection with *L. monocytogenes* whereas this conversion occurs much slower (greater than 6 months) following an acute infection with LCMV (Badovinac and Harty, 2007; Wherry *et al.*, 2003). The differences in memory phenotype progression may be related to differences in cell tropism, pathogen replication cycle, strength of the TCR signal, and the profile of inflammatory cytokines.

Studies from our laboratories have shown that inflammation can dramatically modulate the rate of memory T cell differentiation (Fig. 5.2). Using the advantages afforded by the murine model of listeriosis, we showed that reducing the overall inflammatory milieu can accelerate the acquisition of memory characteristics. We observed that antigen-specific CD8 T cells acquired memory characteristics with enhanced kinetics when *L. monocytogenes* infection was terminated early with antibiotic treatment or when mice were pretreated with antibiotics (Badovinac and Harty, 2007). Importantly, as opposed to what is normally observed following *L. monocytogenes* infection, antigen-specific cells generated in a reduced inflammatory environment could be boosted as early as 2 weeks postinfection (Fig. 5.2) (Badovinac *et al.*, 2005). Interestingly, the acquisition of early memory characteristics, including early acquisition of boostability, was reversed in antibiotic-treated mice in which inflammation was restored by injecting the TLR9 agonist CpG (Fig. 5.2) (Badovinac *et al.*, 2005).

Further, in another study, our laboratories showed that CD8 T cell responses in mice that were pretreated with antibiotics prior to *L. monocytogenes* infection had decreased expansion and contraction phases (Badovinac *et al.*, 2004). These CD8 T cells developed accelerated phenotypic and functional characteristics of memory CD8 T cells including the capacity for vigorous secondary expansion and increased protection of mice from subsequent infection (Badovinac *et al.*, 2004). Similarly, our groups have also demonstrated that vaccination of mice with peptide-coated DCs also results in the acceleration of the memory CD8 T cell pool and that this accelerated memory generation is abrogated in the presence of systemic inflammation induced by CpG treatment (Badovinac *et al.*, 2005; Pham *et al.*, 2009, 2010). Taken together, these results demonstrate that the contraction phase is not necessary for memory progression of

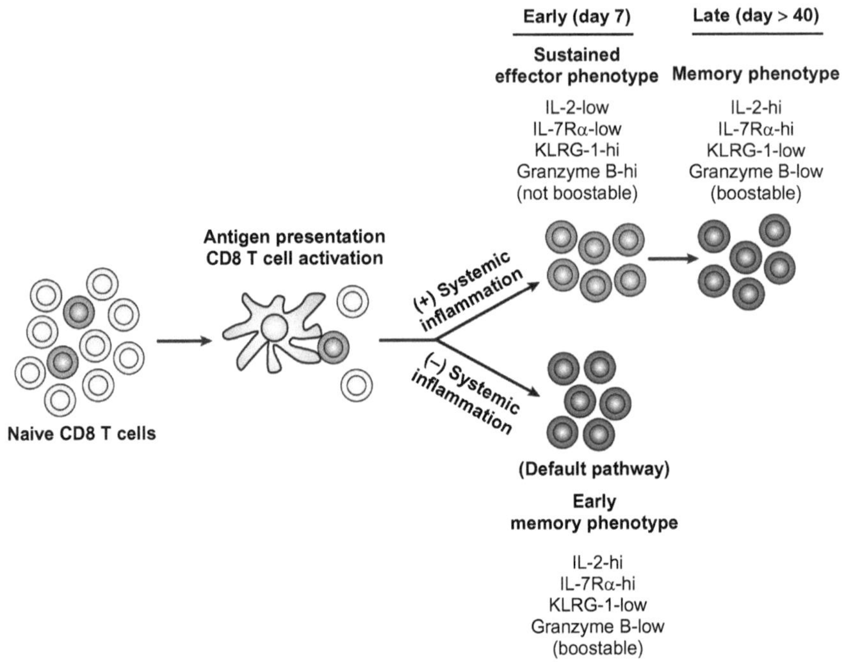

FIGURE 5.2 Inflammation modulates the rate of CD8 T cell memory differentiation. Antigen-specific effector CD8 T cells responding to an infection within a reduced inflammatory environment acquire a memory CD8 T cell phenotype with faster kinetics (IL-2^{hi}, IL-$7R\alpha^{hi}$, KLRG1^{low}, and granzyme B^{low}) and can be boosted earlier than what is normally observed following *L. monocytogenes* infection. Systemic inflammation is required to divert T cells from the default memory pathway and sustain effector functions of responding T cells. (See Color Insert.)

antigen-specific CD8 T cells and that duration of inflammation modulates the rate at which CD8 T cells acquire phenotypic and functional memory characteristics. This may represent an important consideration for the development of effective and rapidly deployable vaccination strategies.

Increasing the numbers of memory CD8 T cells has been directly correlated with increased protection from reinfection (Harty and Badovinac, 2008; Kaech *et al.*, 2002b; Schmidt *et al.*, 2008, 2010). Prime-boost vaccine strategies exploit this in order to generate high numbers of memory cells. This involves priming CD8 T cell responses to a target antigen that are subsequently boosted with the readministration of the same antigen in the context of a different vector (Woodland, 2004). However, due to the inherent difficulty in boosting effector cells, this approach requires several months between each immunization before cells can acquire a memory phenotype and the greatest amplification of memory cells is achieved (Butler *et al.*, 2011a). Thus, reducing the time interval between priming and boosting is desirable, especially in situations when accelerated protection is paramount such as during pandemic infections.

Work from our laboratories has clearly shown that a highly inflamed environment generated by infection or strong adjuvants slows the acquisition memory characteristics by CD8 T cells (Fig. 5.2). Limiting the exposure of antigen-specific CD8 T cells to pro-inflammatory cytokines, as demonstrated with antibiotic-treated mice or peptide-coated DC immunization, results in accelerated acquisition of memory characteristics by responding CD8 T cell. In turn, this allows for optimal booster responses within days postinitial immunization (Badovinac and Harty, 2007; Badovinac *et al.*, 2005; Butler and Harty, 2010; Pham *et al.*, 2009, 2010). These results suggest that, in contrast to strategies that elicit T cell responses with strong adjuvants, prime-boost vaccination strategies could aim to limit systemic inflammation for the priming step. This would likely allow for a rapid boosting of the response shortly after the initial priming. This approach may yield vaccines that can generate the large amounts of memory CD8 T cells required for protection in a short period of time.

4.2. Memory CD8 T cell maintenance

One important characteristic of memory CD8 T cell populations is their capacity to be maintained, at relatively stable numbers for extended periods of time (Homann *et al.*, 2001). Memory CD8 T cells numbers are maintained through a slow homeostatic proliferative process. As such, the numerical stability of memory T cell population suggests that proliferation must be accompanied by an equal rate of memory CD8 T cell death. However, the mechanisms that ensure the balance between proliferation and death of memory T cells required to maintain stable numbers of cells are currently unknown.

Survival and maintenance of memory CD8 T cells does not require TCR signaling but rather depends upon the cytokines IL-7 and IL-15 (Becker *et al.*, 2002; Leignadier *et al.*, 2008; Murali-Krishna *et al.*, 1999; Schluns and Lefrancois, 2003; Schluns *et al.*, 2000). IL-15 signaling plays an important role in the proliferation necessary for the overall maintenance of memory T cells. While memory T cells can be generated in IL-15-deficient hosts, the numbers of memory T cells gradually decline over time. Conversely, IL-7 signaling is important for survival in both naive and memory CD8 T cells (Becker *et al.*, 2002). Further, as described above, IL-7Rα expression has been suggested to mark cells that will eventually survive contraction and form the memory population (Kaech *et al.*, 2003). However, we observed that constitutive expression of IL-7Rα does not confer a survival advantage for responding CD8 T cells (Haring *et al.*, 2008). These results demonstrated that constitutive expression of IL-7Rα does not impair or improve CD8 T cell function, indicating that IL-7Rα alone does not increase survival of effector antigen-specific CD8 T cells and favor the transition into the memory phase. In addition, the generation of antigen-specific effector CD8 T cells remains unaffected at the peak of the response in mice unable to translate some IL-7 mediated signals due to a knock-in mutation in IL-7Rα (IL-7Rα^{449F}) (Osborne *et al.*, 2007). Interestingly, the long-term maintenance of memory CD8 T cells was decreased in these mice indicating the IL-7 mediated signals may generally be more important for the overall maintenance of the memory population. Thus, it is becoming increasingly clear that while IL-7Rα expression may mark cells that eventually survive contraction to become memory cells, expression of this cytokine receptor is not sufficient to favor the development of memory T cell.

4.3. Diversification of memory CD8 T cells upon multiple antigen stimulations

Infection of laboratory mice with *L. monocytogenes* and other model pathogens such as LCMV has generated a wealth of knowledge on the mechanisms of CD8 memory T cell establishment and maintenance. However, while the bulk of our knowledge is centered on memory T cells generated following a single antigenic encounter, humans are often infected multiple times with related pathogens. As such, memory T cell populations resulting from multiple antigen encounters may be common. Further, current vaccination strategies often rely on one or more rounds of booster immunization in order to generate sufficient numbers of memory T cells required to provide protective immunity. It is therefore, imperative to gain a better understanding of the effects of multiple antigenic stimulations on the overall properties of memory CD8 T cells.

Using a combination of an attenuated strain of *L. monocytogenes* expressing OVA and OT-I cells, a recent study from our laboratories determined the impact of multiple antigen encounters on the transcriptional profile of the resulting memory CD8 T cell populations (Wirth *et al.*, 2010). The experimental approach used in this study was based on repeated adoptive transfers of antigen-specific OT-I T cells to naive mice prior to rechallenge with *L. monocytogenes*, thereby allowing for a direct comparison of the transcriptome of memory cells that only differed in their number of antigenic encounters. This approach revealed a potential "core signature" of genes that are differentially regulated between naive and memory T cells but remained shared between memory T cells regardless of the number of antigenic stimulations. Importantly, this included genes that are not currently used to mark memory T cell populations and could therefore lead to the identification of new markers of memory T cells.

This study also revealed a stepwise diversification in the transcriptional profile of memory T cells induced by repeated antigen stimulation (Fig. 5.3A) (Wirth *et al.*, 2010). More than 700 genes were differentially regulated between primary and quaternary memory CD8 T cells and each round of antigenic stimulation was sufficient to differentially regulate a large number of genes. In fact, the number of genes differentially regulated following each additional round of antigenic stimulation was nearly equivalent to the number of genes that are differentially regulated between naive and primary memory CD8 T cells. This demonstrated that repeated antigen stimulation continually drives the diversification in gene expression in memory CD8 T cells and revealed a previously unappreciated level of heterogeneity amongst the memory CD8 T cell pool.

Of particular interest, direct comparison of primary and quaternary memory presenting with a T_{EM} phenotype still revealed significant differences in gene expression profiles, strongly suggesting that multiple antigenic stimulation induces heterogeneity that may go well beyond the classical T_{CM} and T_{EM} classifications (Wirth *et al.*, 2010). Repeated antigenic stimulation resulted in transcription changes of genes from multiple gene families including genes involved in T cell trafficking, effector functions, metabolism, cell cycle regulation, and signal transduction (Fig. 5.3B and C). Interestingly, several transcription factors were observed to maintain a stepwise increase or decrease in transcription levels with each additional antigen stimulation, suggesting that these transcription factors may play a critical role in the progressive diversification in gene expression of memory CD8 T cell populations. The transcription profile generated over the course of these experiments represents a list of potential targets that can be manipulated to directly understand their function in memory T cells. Gaining a better understanding of what role these and other differentially regulated genes play in the biology and function of multiply stimulated memory T cell will likely provide critical information for the design of effective prime-boost vaccination strategies.

One important difference between primary memory and multiply stimulated memory T cells is the maintenance of an effector-like phenotype. Each round of antigen stimulation progressively delays reacquisition of surface expression of CD62L and CCR7 and progressively reduces the capacity of these cells to produce IL-2 (Fig. 5.3B) (Jabbari and Harty, 2006; Masopust *et al.*, 2006; Nolz and Harty, 2011; Wirth *et al.*, 2010). Delayed capacity to acquire central memory-like characteristics has been suggested to relate to changes in the homeostatic proliferative potential of these cells, a change that can in part be explained by the progressive decline in surface expression of cytokine receptors such as IL-2/IL-15Rβ following each round of antigenic stimulation (Jabbari and Harty, 2006). Consistent with these changes in the expression of lymph node homing markers, multiply stimulated memory CD8 T cells preferentially accumulate in

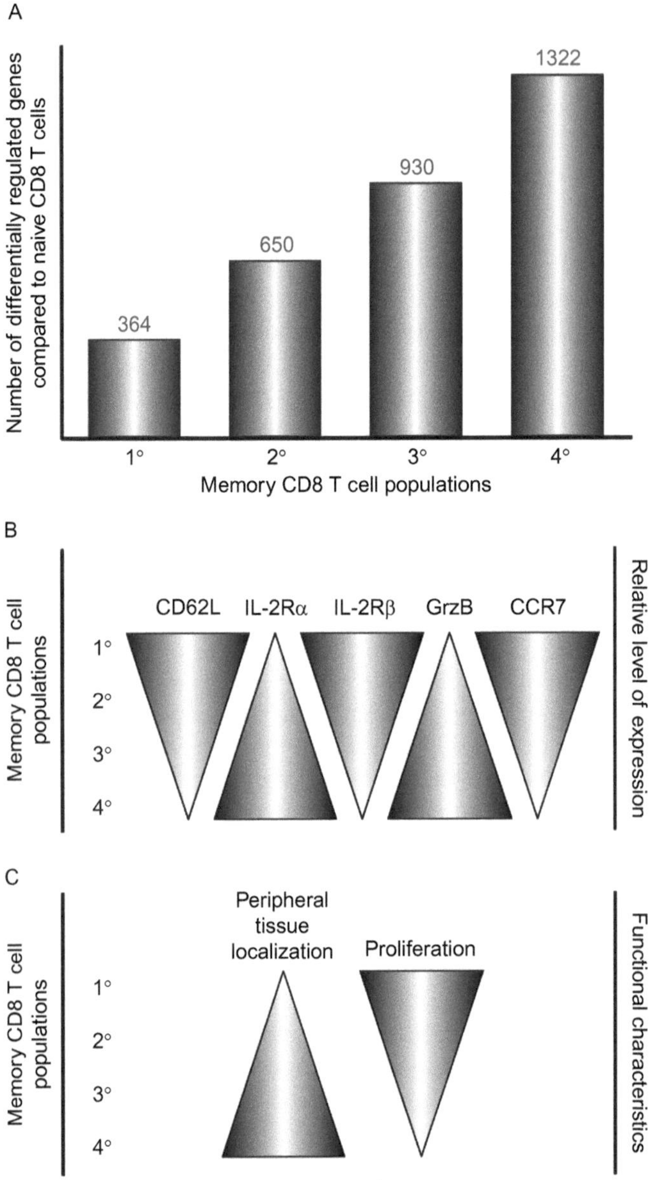

FIGURE 5.3 Repeated antigenic encounters have a progressive impact on the molecular signature of memory CD8 T cells. The transcriptome of memory CD8 T cells was compared based on their number of antigenic encounters by repeated adoptive transfers of antigen-specific OT-I cells into naive mice prior to rechallenge with *L. monocytogenes* (Wirth *et al.*, 2010). (A) Compared to naive CD8 T cells, primary (1°) and repeatedly stimulated (secondary (2°), tertiary (3°), and quaternary (4°)) memory CD8 T

peripheral tissues (Fig. 5.3C) (Jabbari and Harty, 2006; Masopust *et al.*, 2006; Nolz and Harty, 2012).

In addition, multiply stimulated cells express higher levels of effector molecules such as granzyme B and display increased capacity to kill target cells *in vivo* (Fig. 5.3B; Jabbari and Harty, 2006; Wirth *et al.*, 2010). Interestingly, these differences in localization and effector function have been demonstrated to affect the capacity of memory T cells to respond to certain infections. Due in part to their preferentially peripheral localization, secondary memory T cells have been demonstrated to be more protective than primary memory T cells against acute infection such as LCMV Armstrong or *L. monocytogenes* (Jabbari and Harty, 2006; Nolz and Harty, 2011). Secondary memory T cells were also demonstrated to allow for increased priming of new antigenic-specific naive T cells, a phenomenon that may have important consequence for the renewal of a memory population (Jabbari and Harty, 2006). However, this scenario is reversed in the case of chronic LCMV infection where secondary memory T cells were recently demonstrated to be significantly less effective at controlling infection (Nolz and Harty, 2011). As primary memory T cells genetically manipulated to prevent lymph node homing similarly lost their protective capacity during chronic infections, the loss of protective capacity in secondary memory T cells appears directly related to their decreased capacity for lymph node homing. Interestingly, secondary memory cells were also observed to be more likely to become functionally exhausted following LCMV clone 13 infections than primary memory cells. These findings have important implications for the design of vaccines aimed at preventing chronic infections particularly for pathogens such as human immunodeficiency virus (HIV) where the virus is known to undergo replication within lymph nodes.

The increased sensitivity of secondary memory T cells to functional exhaustion over the course of chronic infection represents an important consideration for prime-boost vaccine strategies. This may be of particular importance in light of the demonstration that repeated antigen

cells have a stepwise diversification upon each additional antigen exposure. Numbers on the graph represent the numbers of genes differentially regulated compared to naive CD8 T cells. (B) Repeated antigenic exposure progressively changes the phenotype of responding CD8 T cells. Each round of antigenic stimulation delays the reacquisition of surface expression of CD62L and CCR7. Additionally, there is a progressive decline in surface expression of cytokine receptors such as IL-2Rβ. Conversely, multiply stimulated cells have increased expression of cytokine receptors such as IL-2Rα and express higher levels of effector molecules such as granzyme B (GrzB). (C) Multiply stimulated memory CD8 T cells preferentially accumulate in peripheral tissues and demonstrate significantly reduced proliferative capacities (i.e., antigen-driven expansion and homeostatic proliferation).

stimulation may generate memory T cells with a terminally differentiated phenotype. Multiply stimulated memory T cells demonstrate significantly reduced proliferative capacities and express lower levels of several genes within the ribosomal pathway, suggesting some level of transcriptional or translational impairment in these cells (Wirth *et al.*, 2010). These two hallmarks have also been described for cells having undergone functional exhaustion (Wherry *et al.*, 2007). In fact, while several genes were differentially expressed, nearly one-third of genes associated with functional exhaustion were also enriched in quaternary memory CD8 T cells (Wirth *et al.*, 2010). Taken together, these data suggest that the potential increase in exhaustibility of multiply stimulated memory cells will need to be taken into consideration when designing vaccine aimed at preventing chronic infection such as those caused by HIV and hepatitis C virus infections.

Another important difference between primary and multiply stimulated memory T cells may relate to their maintenance and their dependence upon certain cytokines for survival. In particular, the expression levels of some cytokine receptor chains such as IL-2Rα and IL-18R1 were increased in multiply stimulated memory cells (Fig. 5.3B) (Wirth *et al.*, 2010). Conversely, transcription levels of IL-2/15Rβ were steadily decreased compared to primary memory with each subsequent round of antigenic stimulation (Fig. 5.3B). Taken together, these data strongly suggest that repeated antigenic stimulations alter the cytokine responsiveness of memory CD8 T cells. Changes in IL-2/15Rβ expression may be of particular interest as this receptor is required for IL-15 signaling, a cytokine that plays a well-described role in the maintenance of primary memory T cells (Becker *et al.*, 2002). Interestingly, a study from our laboratory has demonstrated that reduced responsiveness to IL-15 may directly explain the slower acquisition of central memory characteristics by secondary memory cells. Specifically, high-dose IL-15 treatment *in vitro* was sufficient to induce proliferation of secondary memory T cells and this correlated with the appearance of cells expressing high levels of CD62L (Jabbari and Harty, 2006). Thus, we could envision the development of strategies aimed at manipulating multiply stimulated memory cells in order to restore their capacity to respond to infections, such as HIV, that require priming within the lymph nodes.

The use of the *L. monocytogenes* murine model has significantly increased our knowledge of the biology of memory CD8 T cells that have encountered multiple rounds of antigenic stimulation. The transcriptional profile of multiply stimulated memory T cells represents an important starting point for future studies aimed at further understanding the properties of these cells. In turn, these studies should generate critical information that may allow for the optimization of prime-boost vaccination strategies.

5. SURROGATE MARKERS TO TRACK ANTIGEN-SPECIFIC CD8 T CELL RESPONSES

The identification of specific CD8 T cell epitopes and the generation of *L. monocytogenes* strains expressing model antigens have significantly contributed to shaping our knowledge of CD8 T responses following infection. Taking advantage of these well-defined epitopes, a study from our laboratories has recently demonstrated that CD8 T cells responding to antigen stimulation *in vivo* exhibit a specific phenotypic footprint (Rai *et al.*, 2009). This can be used to identify responding T cells without *a priori* knowledge of specific epitopes or MHC molecules used to present these epitopes.

Following challenge with *L. monocytogenes* expressing OVA, CD8 T cells specific for the OVA epitope downregulated surface expression of CD8α and upregulated the expression of the integrin molecule CD11a. Importantly, these phenotypic changes are controlled by antigen stimulation rather than by systemic inflammation, as OT-I cells did not exhibit these phenotypic changes when mice were injected with TLR agonists or challenged with an *L. monocytogenes* strain that does not express OVA. Further, these changes are maintained in a variety of tissues and are stable such that they can also be used to track memory T cell responses. Thus, this surrogate marker approach can be used to track antigen-specific T cells without any *a priori* knowledge of their specificity.

This approach has already been used to study responses in outbred mouse strains revealing a previously unappreciated level of host-to-host variability in CD8 T cell responses to a single pathogen (Rai *et al.*, 2009). Perhaps more importantly, this technique has also allowed for studies of the CD8 T cell response in other highly relevant pathogens such as *Plasmodium*, the causative agent of malaria. More specifically, using this technique our laboratory has been able to study some of the functional and numerical requirements for protective CD8 T cell responses following immunization with attenuated sporozoites (Butler *et al.*, 2011b; Schmidt *et al.*, 2010). This approach is likely to further our understanding of CD8 T cell responses to a variety of other important pathogens and is likely to significantly impact our approach to vaccine development.

6. FUTURE DIRECTIONS

6.1. *L. monocytogenes* as a model for mucosal CD8 T cell responses

Although intravenous infection with *L. monocytogenes* has significantly increased our understanding of all phases of the CD8 T cells response following infection, little is known about the CD8 T cell responses induced following *L. monocytogenes* entry via natural oral route of infection. This is primarily due to the fact that *L. monocytogenes* is poorly able to infect laboratory mice through the oral route (Lecuit, 2007). While other animal models such as ferrets and hamsters are naturally permissive to oral infection with *L. monocytogenes*, the "toolbox" for studying CD8 T cell responses in these models is not as well developed rendering studies much more challenging (Lecuit, 2007).

The disparities in susceptibility to oral infection are dictated by differences in E-cadherin, a molecule that plays a critical role in internalization of the bacteria. Interestingly, the inability of murine E-cadherin to mediate bacterial entry depends on a single amino acid at position 16, which is a proline in permissive hosts such as humans and a glutamic acid residue in nonpermissive rats and mice (Lecuit *et al.*, 1999). This discovery has led to the development of transgenic mouse models where expression of murine E-cadherin is replaced by human E-cadherin strictly within enterocytes. These modifications were sufficient to render mice highly susceptible to oral infection with *L. monocytogenes* (Lecuit *et al.*, 2001). This model and any derivative that can be generated by crossing these mice to other gene-deficient mice of interest is likely to generate wealth of data regarding the CD8 T cell responses induced by bacterial infections at mucosal surfaces. This may allow for all the inherent advantages of the murine model of listeriosis to be harnessed for the study of mucosal CD8 T cell responses. This increased knowledge of the biology of mucosal CD8 T cell responses is, in turn, likely to advance our knowledge of the requirements for protection against other important mucosal pathogens such as influenza A or HIV.

6.2. *L. monocytogenes* as a live vaccine vector

One major challenge to developing effective vaccine has always been the generation of safe, effective vectors to carry antigens of interest. Enteric bacterial vectors represent a potentially promising vaccine strategy. They are relatively inexpensive to make and highly attenuated strains can be generated that can be safely used in immunocompromised individuals. Additionally, they can be engineered to be sensitive to antibiotic, thus providing treatment options in case adverse reactions occur, and can easily be administered orally. *L. monocytogenes*' ability to reproducibly induce potent CD8 T cell responses has prompted its development as a potential vaccine vector.

To address these safety concerns, different aspects of the bacterial life cycle have been targeted to generate mutant *L. monocytogenes* strains that are attenuated from wild-type strains. LLO-deficient *L. monocytogenes* strains, which cannot escape the phagosome, are highly attenuated and some studies suggest that they may not elicit protective immunity (Barry *et al.*, 1992; Berche *et al.*, 1987). However, work from our laboratories has shown that infection with LLO-deficient *L. monocytogenes* strains results in the induction of a CD8 T cell response that is protective against secondary challenge (Hamilton *et al.*, 2006). Further, using this attenuated bacterial vector, it was demonstrated that CD8 T cells could be primed against endogenous or recombinant antigens resulting in the establishment of a functional memory CD8 T cell population. Additionally, while lowering the dose by as much as 1000-fold resulted in undetectable primary antigen-specific CD8 T cells, these mice were still able to mount an enhanced response to early booster immunization. These results are important and demonstrate that cytosolic entry is not required to develop protective CD8 T cell responses illustrating the potential of utilizing highly attenuated *L. monocytogenes* strains for vaccine strategies.

Other approaches have been used to yield highly attenuated *L. monocytogenes* strains. Remarkably, one of these strains (Lmdd, lacking two genes for D-alanine synthesis) was demonstrated to have dramatically reduced pathogenicity even in neonatal mice and has been further shown to be safe even at high doses in feeding trials of macaques (Lieberman and Frankel, 2002). Additionally, these strains have been engineered to express HIV proteins and as such may represent a potentially important development in the search for an effective HIV vaccine and trials to this effect are currently underway (Jiang *et al.*, 2007; Lakhashe *et al.*, 2011; Lieberman and Frankel, 2002; Zhao *et al.*, 2006). In addition, a new class of killed but metabolically active *L. monocytogenes* vaccine vectors has recently been described. These vectors are based on the photochemical inactivation of bacterial mutants lacking nucleotide excision repair capacities. This approach has been demonstrated to elicit protective CD8 T cell responses in mice and may represent a potential new avenue for vaccine development (Brockstedt *et al.*, 2005).

One consideration for utilizing attenuated recombinant *L. monocytogenes* strains as a vaccine vector is whether immunity to the vector itself affects the effectiveness of the vaccine (Leong *et al.*, 2009; Martin *et al.*, 2011). During the initial infection or immunization, not all of the antigen-specific naive CD8 T cells are recruited into the response resulting in an environment where antigen-specific naive and memory CD8 T cells coexist. Recently, our laboratories have investigated the impact of preexisting memory CD8 T cells on newly recruited naive CD8 T cells (Martin *et al.*, 2011). This study demonstrated that existing anti-vectorial memory CD8 T cells influence naive CD8 T cell response. Naive CD8 T cells primed in the presence of memory developed accelerated phenotypic and functional characteristics of memory CD8 T cells compared to naive CD8 T cells primed in a nonimmune environment. These results have important implications for rationale vaccine strategies, illustrating that anti-vectorial immunity may have an effect on newly generated memory CD8 T cells, thus providing insight into designing effective vaccines.

7. CONCLUSION

Infection of laboratory mice with *L. monocytogenes* has contributed tremendously to our current knowledge of all facets of CD8 T cell biology. This remarkable bacterium continues to be a workhorse for CD8 T cell biologists and is likely to continue to advance our knowledge of CD8 T cell responses for years to come. The many advantages of this system, including the generation of attenuated and recombinant strains, have allowed for many seminal discoveries that have greatly advanced our knowledge of CD8 T cell responses to infection. Importantly, the findings drawn from this model are likely to continue to have broad implications for our knowledge of responses to other pathogens and to allow for continuing improvements in the development of effective vaccine strategies.

ACKNOWLEDGMENTS

The authors would like to acknowledge former and current members of the Badovinac and Harty laboratories for their contributions to this work. We also offer apologies to the many investigators whose contribution we were unable to discuss owing to space limitations. Work described in this review was supported by grants from the NIH: AI36864, AI46653, AI42767, AI50073, AI059752, AI85515 (J. T. H.), and AI83286 (V. P. B.). M. J. R. is supported by a fellowship from the Canadian Institutes of Health Research.

REFERENCES

Aichele, P., Unsoeld, H., Koschella, M., Schweier, O., Kalinke, U., and Vucikuja, S. (2006). CD8 T cells specific for lymphocytic choriomeningitis virus require type I IFN receptor for clonal expansion. *J. Immunol.* **176,** 4525.

Badovinac, V. P., and Harty, J. T. (2002). CD8(+) T-cell homeostasis after infection: Setting the 'curve'. *Microbes Infect.* **4,** 441.

Badovinac, V. P., and Harty, J. T. (2006). Programming, demarcating, and manipulating CD8+ T-cell memory. *Immunol. Rev.* **211,** 67.

Badovinac, V. P., and Harty, J. T. (2007). Manipulating the rate of memory CD8+ T cell generation after acute infection. *J. Immunol.* **179,** 53.

Badovinac, V. P., Tvinnereim, A. R., and Harty, J. T. (2000). Regulation of antigen-specific CD8+ T cell homeostasis by perforin and interferon-gamma. *Science* **290,** 1354.

Badovinac, V. P., Porter, B. B., and Harty, J. T. (2002). Programmed contraction of CD8(+) T cells after infection. *Nat. Immunol.* **3,** 619.

Badovinac, V. P., Porter, B. B., and Harty, J. T. (2004). CD8+ T cell contraction is controlled by early inflammation. *Nat. Immunol.* **5,** 809.

Badovinac, V. P., Messingham, K. A., Jabbari, A., Haring, J. S., and Harty, J. T. (2005). Accelerated CD8+ T-cell memory and prime-boost response after dendritic-cell vaccination. *Nat. Med.* **11,** 748.

Bancroft, G. J., Sheehan, K. C., Schreiber, R. D., and Unanue, E. R. (1989). Tumor necrosis factor is involved in the T cell-independent pathway of macrophage activation in scid mice. *J. Immunol.* **143,** 127.

Barry, R. A., Bouwer, H. G., Portnoy, D. A., and Hinrichs, D. J. (1992). Pathogenicity and immunogenicity of Listeria monocytogenes small-plaque mutants defective for intracellular growth and cell-to-cell spread. *Infect. Immun.* **60,** 1625.

Becker, T. C., Wherry, E. J., Boone, D., Murali-Krishna, K., Antia, R., Ma, A., and Ahmed, R. (2002). Interleukin 15 is required for proliferative renewal of virus-specific memory CD8 T cells. *J. Exp. Med.* **195,** 1541.

Berche, P., Gaillard, J. L., and Sansonetti, P. J. (1987). Intracellular growth of Listeria monocytogenes as a prerequisite for in vivo induction of T cell-mediated immunity. *J. Immunol.* **138,** 2266.

Bevan, M. J. (2004). Helping the CD8(+) T-cell response. *Nat. Rev. Immunol.* **4,** 595.

Blattman, J. N., Antia, R., Sourdive, D. J., Wang, X., Kaech, S. M., Murali-Krishna, K., Altman, J. D., and Ahmed, R. (2002). Estimating the precursor frequency of naive antigen-specific CD8 T cells. *J. Exp. Med.* **195,** 657.

Brockstedt, D. G., Bahjat, K. S., Giedlin, M. A., Liu, W., Leong, M., Luckett, W., Gao, Y., Schnupf, P., Kapadia, D., Castro, G., Lim, J. Y., Sampson-Johannes, A., *et al.* (2005). Killed but metabolically active microbes: A new vaccine paradigm for eliciting effector T-cell responses and protective immunity. *Nat. Med.* **11,** 853.

Buchmeier, N. A., and Schreiber, R. D. (1985). Requirement of endogenous interferon-gamma production for resolution of Listeria monocytogenes infection. *Proc. Natl. Acad. Sci. USA* **82,** 7404.

Busch, D. H., Pilip, I. M., Vijh, S., and Pamer, E. G. (1998). Coordinate regulation of complex T cell populations responding to bacterial infection. *Immunity* **8,** 353.

Butler, N. S., and Harty, J. T. (2010). The role of inflammation in the generation and maintenance of memory T cells. *Adv. Exp. Med. Biol.* **684,** 42.

Butler, N. S., Nolz, J. C., and Harty, J. T. (2011a). Immunologic considerations for generating memory CD8 T cells through vaccination. *Cell. Microbiol.* **13,** 925.

Butler, N. S., Schmidt, N. W., Vaughan, A. M., Aly, A. S., Kappe, S. H., and Harty, J. T. (2011b). Superior antimalarial immunity after vaccination with late liver stage-arresting genetically attenuated parasites. *Cell Host Microbe* **9,** 451.

Butz, E. A., and Bevan, M. J. (1998). Massive expansion of antigen-specific CD8+ T cells during an acute virus infection. *Immunity* **8,** 167.

Casrouge, A., Beaudoing, E., Dalle, S., Pannetier, C., Kanellopoulos, J., and Kourilsky, P. (2000). Size estimate of the alpha beta TCR repertoire of naive mouse splenocytes. *J. Immunol.* **164,** 5782.

Corbin, G. A., and Harty, J. T. (2004). Duration of infection and antigen display have minimal influence on the kinetics of the CD4+ T cell response to Listeria monocytogenes infection. *J. Immunol.* **173,** 5679.

Curtsinger, J. M., and Mescher, M. F. (2010). Inflammatory cytokines as a third signal for T cell activation. *Curr. Opin. Immunol.* **22,** 333.

Curtsinger, J. M., Schmidt, C. S., Mondino, A., Lins, D. C., Kedl, R. M., Jenkins, M. K., and Mescher, M. F. (1999). Inflammatory cytokines provide a third signal for activation of naive CD4+ and CD8+ T cells. *J. Immunol.* **162,** 3256.

Curtsinger, J. M., Johnson, C. M., and Mescher, M. F. (2003). CD8 T cell clonal expansion and development of effector function require prolonged exposure to antigen, costimulation, and signal 3 cytokine. *J. Immunol.* **171,** 5165.

Fruh, K., and Yang, Y. (1999). Antigen presentation by MHC class I and its regulation by interferon gamma. *Curr. Opin. Immunol.* **11,** 76.

Fuller, M. J., Khanolkar, A., Tebo, A. E., and Zajac, A. J. (2004). Maintenance, loss, and resurgence of T cell responses during acute, protracted, and chronic viral infections. *J. Immunol.* **172,** 4204.

Hamilton, S. E., Badovinac, V. P., Khanolkar, A., and Harty, J. T. (2006). Listeriolysin O-deficient Listeria monocytogenes as a vaccine delivery vehicle: Antigen-specific CD8 T cell priming and protective immunity. *J. Immunol.* **177,** 4012.

Hamon, M., Bierne, H., and Cossart, P. (2006). Listeria monocytogenes: A multifaceted model. *Nat. Rev. Microbiol.* **4,** 423.

Hand, T. W., Morre, M., and Kaech, S. M. (2007). Expression of IL-7 receptor alpha is necessary but not sufficient for the formation of memory CD8 T cells during viral infection. *Proc. Natl. Acad. Sci. USA* **104**(28),11730–11735.

Haring, J. S., Jing, X., Bollenbacher-Reilley, J., Xue, H. H., Leonard, W. J., and Harty, J. T. (2008). Constitutive expression of IL-7 receptor alpha does not support increased expansion or prevent contraction of antigen-specific CD4 or CD8 T cells following Listeria monocytogenes infection. *J. Immunol.* **180,** 2855.

Harty, J. T., and Badovinac, V. P. (2002). Influence of effector molecules on the CD8(+) T cell response to infection. *Curr. Opin. Immunol.* **14,** 360.

Harty, J. T., and Badovinac, V. P. (2008). Shaping and reshaping CD8+ T-cell memory. *Nat. Rev. Immunol.* **8,** 107.

Harty, J. T., and Bevan, M. J. (1995). Specific immunity to Listeria monocytogenes in the absence of IFN gamma. *Immunity* **3,** 109.

Harty, J. T., and Bevan, M. J. (1999). Responses of CD8(+) T cells to intracellular bacteria. *Curr. Opin. Immunol.* **11,** 89.

Harty, J. T., Tvinnereim, A. R., and White, D. W. (2000). CD8+ T cell effector mechanisms in resistance to infection. *Annu. Rev. Immunol.* **18,** 275.

Havenar-Daughton, C., Kolumam, G. A., and Murali-Krishna, K. (2006). Cutting Edge: The direct action of type I IFN on CD4 T cells is critical for sustaining clonal expansion in response to a viral but not a bacterial infection. *J. Immunol.* **176,** 3315.

Hogquist, K. A., Jameson, S. C., Heath, W. R., Howard, J. L., Bevan, M. J., and Carbone, F. R. (1994). T cell receptor antagonist peptides induce positive selection. *Cell* **76,** 17.

Homann, D., Teyton, L., and Oldstone, M. B. (2001). Differential regulation of antiviral T-cell immunity results in stable CD8+ but declining CD4+ T-cell memory. *Nat. Med.* **7,** 913.

Huang, S., Hendriks, W., Althage, A., Hemmi, S., Bluethmann, H., Kamijo, R., Vilcek, J., Zinkernagel, R. M., and Aguet, M. (1993). Immune response in mice that lack the interferon-gamma receptor. *Science* **259,** 1742.

Jabbari, A., and Harty, J. T. (2006). Secondary memory CD8+ T cells are more protective but slower to acquire a central-memory phenotype. *J. Exp. Med.* **203,** 919.

Jameson, S. C., and Masopust, D. (2009). Diversity in T cell memory: An embarrassment of riches. *Immunity* **31,** 859.

Jiang, S., Rasmussen, R. A., Nolan, K. M., Frankel, F. R., Lieberman, J., McClure, H. M., Williams, K. M., Babu, U. S., Raybourne, R. B., Strobert, E., and Ruprecht, R. M. (2007). Live attenuated Listeria monocytogenes expressing HIV Gag: Immunogenicity in rhesus monkeys. *Vaccine* **25,** 7470.

Kaech, S. M., and Ahmed, R. (2001). Memory CD8+ T cell differentiation: Initial antigen encounter triggers a developmental program in naive cells. *Nat. Immunol.* **2,** 415.

Kaech, S. M., Hemby, S., Kersh, E., and Ahmed, R. (2002a). Molecular and functional profiling of memory CD8 T cell differentiation. *Cell* **111,** 837.

Kaech, S. M., Wherry, E. J., and Ahmed, R. (2002b). Effector and memory T-cell differentiation: Implications for vaccine development. *Nat. Rev. Immunol.* **2,** 251.

Kaech, S. M., Tan, J. T., Wherry, E. J., Konieczny, B. T., Surh, C. D., and Ahmed, R. (2003). Selective expression of the interleukin 7 receptor identifies effector CD8 T cells that give rise to long-lived memory cells. *Nat. Immunol.* **4,** 1191.

Kagi, D., Odermatt, B., and Mak, T. W. (1999). Homeostatic regulation of CD8+ T cells by perforin. *Eur. J. Immunol.* **29,** 3262.

Kolumam, G. A., Thomas, S., Thompson, L. J., Sprent, J., and Murali-Krishna, K. (2005). Type I interferons act directly on CD8 T cells to allow clonal expansion and memory formation in response to viral infection. *J. Exp. Med.* **202,** 637.

Lacombe, M. H., Hardy, M. P., Rooney, J., and Labrecque, N. (2005). IL-7 receptor expression levels do not identify CD8+ memory T lymphocyte precursors following peptide immunization. *J. Immunol.* **175,** 4400.

Lakhashe, S. K., Velu, V., Sciaranghella, G., Siddappa, N. B., Dipasquale, J. M., Hemashettar, G., Yoon, J. K., Rasmussen, R. A., Yang, F., Lee, S. J., Montefiori, D. C., Novembre, F. J., *et al.* (2011). Prime-boost vaccination with heterologous live vectors encoding SIV gag and multimeric HIV-1 gp160 protein: Efficacy against repeated mucosal R5 clade C SHIV challenges. *Vaccine* **29,** 5611.

Lara-Tejero, M., and Pamer, E. G. (2004). T cell responses to Listeria monocytogenes. *Curr. Opin. Microbiol.* **7,** 45.

Lecuit, M. (2007). Human listeriosis and animal models. *Microbes Infect.* **9,** 1216.

Lecuit, M., Dramsi, S., Gottardi, C., Fedor-Chaiken, M., Gumbiner, B., and Cossart, P. (1999). A single amino acid in E-cadherin responsible for host specificity towards the human pathogen Listeria monocytogenes. *EMBO J.* **18,** 3956.

Lecuit, M., Vandormael-Pournin, S., Lefort, J., Huerre, M., Gounon, P., Dupuy, C., Babinet, C., and Cossart, P. (2001). A transgenic model for listeriosis: Role of internalin in crossing the intestinal barrier. *Science* **292,** 1722.

Leignadier, J., Hardy, M. P., Cloutier, M., Rooney, J., and Labrecque, N. (2008). Memory T-lymphocyte survival does not require T-cell receptor expression. *Proc. Natl. Acad. Sci. USA* **105,** 20440.

Leong, M. L., Hampl, J., Liu, W., Mathur, S., Bahjat, K. S., Luckett, W., Dubensky, T. W., Jr., and Brockstedt, D. G. (2009). Impact of preexisting vector-specific immunity on vaccine potency: Characterization of Listeria monocytogenes-specific humoral and cellular immunity in humans and modeling studies using recombinant vaccines in mice. *Infect. Immun.* **77,** 3958.

Lieberman, J., and Frankel, F. R. (2002). Engineered Listeria monocytogenes as an AIDS vaccine. *Vaccine* **20,** 2007.

Mackaness, G. B. (1962). Cellular resistance to infection. *J. Exp. Med.* **116,** 381.

Mackaness, G. B. (1964). Immunological basis of acquired cellular resistance. *J. Exp. Med.* **120,** 105.

Marrack, P., Kappler, J., and Mitchell, T. (1999). Type I interferons keep activated T cells alive. *J. Exp. Med.* **189,** 521.

Martin, M. D., Wirth, T. C., Lauer, P., Harty, J. T., and Badovinac, V. P. (2011). The impact of pre-existing memory on differentiation of newly recruited naive CD8 T cells. *J. Immunol.* **187,** 2923–2931.

Masopust, D., Vezys, V., Marzo, A. L., and Lefrancois, L. (2001). Preferential localization of effector memory cells in nonlymphoid tissue. *Science* **291,** 2413.

Masopust, D., Ha, S. J., Vezys, V., and Ahmed, R. (2006). Stimulation history dictates memory CD8 T cell phenotype: Implications for prime-boost vaccination. *J. Immunol.* **177,** 831.

Matloubian, M., Suresh, M., Glass, A., Galvan, M., Chow, K., Whitmire, J. K., Walsh, C. M., Clark, W. R., and Ahmed, R. (1999). A role for perforin in downregulating T-cell responses during chronic viral infection. *J. Virol.* **73,** 2527.

Mercado, R., Vijh, S., Allen, S. E., Kerksiek, K., Pilip, I. M., and Pamer, E. G. (2000). Early programming of T cell populations responding to bacterial infection. *J. Immunol.* **165,** 6833.

Moon, J. J., Chu, H. H., Pepper, M., McSorley, S. J., Jameson, S. C., Kedl, R. M., and Jenkins, M. K. (2007). Naive CD4(+) T cell frequency varies for different epitopes and predicts repertoire diversity and response magnitude. *Immunity* **27,** 203.

Morgan, D. J., Liblau, R., Scott, B., Fleck, S., McDevitt, H. O., Sarvetnick, N., Lo, D., and Sherman, L. A. (1996). CD8(+) T cell-mediated spontaneous diabetes in neonatal mice. *J. Immunol.* **157,** 978.

Murali-Krishna, K., Altman, J. D., Suresh, M., Sourdive, D. J., Zajac, A. J., Miller, J. D., Slansky, J., and Ahmed, R. (1998). Counting antigen-specific CD8 T cells: A reevaluation of bystander activation during viral infection. *Immunity* **8,** 177.

Murali-Krishna, K., Lau, L. L., Sambhara, S., Lemonnier, F., Altman, J., and Ahmed, R. (1999). Persistence of memory CD8 T cells in MHC class I-deficient mice. *Science* **286,** 1377.

Murray, E. G. D., Webb, R. A., and Swann, M. B. R. (1926). A disease of rabbits characterised by a large mononuclear leucocytosis, caused by a hitherto undescribed bacillus Bacterium monocytogenes (n.sp.). *J. Pathol. Bacteriol.* **29,** 407.

Nolz, J. C., and Harty, J. T. (2011). Protective capacity of memory CD8+ T cells is dictated by antigen exposure history and nature of the infection. *Immunity* **34,** 781.

Nolz, J. C., and Harty, J. T. (2012). Strategies and implications for prime-boost vaccination to generate memory CD8 T Cells. *Adv. Exp. Med. Biol.* **780,** 69.

Obar, J. J., Khanna, K. M., and Lefrancois, L. (2008). Endogenous naive CD8+ T cell precursor frequency regulates primary and memory responses to infection. *Immunity* **28,** 859.

Osborne, L. C., Dhanji, S., Snow, J. W., Priatel, J. J., Ma, M. C., Miners, M. J., Teh, H. S., Goldsmith, M. A., and Abraham, N. (2007). Impaired CD8 T cell memory and CD4 T cell primary responses in IL-7R alpha mutant mice. *J. Exp. Med.* **204,** 619.

Pamer, E. G. (1994). Direct sequence identification and kinetic analysis of an MHC class I-restricted Listeria monocytogenes CTL epitope. *J. Immunol.* **152,** 686.

Pamer, E. G. (2004). Immune responses to Listeria monocytogenes. *Nat. Rev. Immunol.* **4,** 812.

Pamer, E. G., Harty, J. T., and Bevan, M. J. (1991). Precise prediction of a dominant class I MHC-restricted epitope of Listeria monocytogenes. *Nature* **353,** 852.

Pearce, E. L., and Shen, H. (2007). Generation of CD8 T cell memory is regulated by IL-12. *J. Immunol.* **179,** 2074.

Pellegrini, M., Belz, G., Bouillet, P., and Strasser, A. (2003). Shutdown of an acute T cell immune response to viral infection is mediated by the proapoptotic Bcl-2 homology 3-only protein Bim. *Proc. Natl. Acad. Sci. USA* **100,** 14175.

Pham, N. L., Badovinac, V. P., and Harty, J. T. (2009). A default pathway of memory CD8 T cell differentiation after dendritic cell immunization is deflected by encounter with inflammatory cytokines during antigen-driven proliferation. *J. Immunol.* **183,** 2337.

Pham, N. L., Pewe, L. L., Fleenor, C. J., Langlois, R. A., Legge, K. L., Badovinac, V. P., and Harty, J. T. (2010). Exploiting cross-priming to generate protective CD8 T-cell immunity rapidly. *Proc. Natl. Acad. Sci. USA* **107,** 12198.

Pham, N. L., Badovinac, V. P., and Harty, J. T. (2011). Differential role of "signal 3" inflammatory cytokines in regulating CD8 T cell expansion and differentiation in vivo. *Front. Immunol.* **2,** 1.

Phillips, T., Opferman, J. T., Shah, R., Liu, N., Froelich, C. J., and Ashton-Rickardt, P. G. (2004). A role for the granzyme B inhibitor serine protease inhibitor 6 in CD8+ memory cell homeostasis. *J. Immunol.* **173,** 3801.

Pircher, H., Baenziger, J., Schilham, M., Sado, T., Kamisaku, H., Hengartner, H., and Zinkernagel, R. M. (1987). Characterization of virus-specific cytotoxic T cell clones from allogeneic bone marrow chimeras. *Eur. J. Immunol.* **17,** 159.

Pope, C., Kim, S. K., Marzo, A., Masopust, D., Williams, K., Jiang, J., Shen, H., and Lefrancois, L. (2001). Organ-specific regulation of the CD8 T cell response to Listeria monocytogenes infection. *J. Immunol.* **166,** 3402.

Porter, B. B., and Harty, J. T. (2006). The onset of CD8+–T-cell contraction is influenced by the peak of Listeria monocytogenes infection and antigen display. *Infect. Immun.* **74,** 1528.

Prlic, M., and Bevan, M. J. (2008). Exploring regulatory mechanisms of CD8+ T cell contraction. *Proc. Natl. Acad. Sci. USA* **105,** 16689.

Rai, D., Pham, N. L., Harty, J. T., and Badovinac, V. P. (2009). Tracking the total CD8 T cell response to infection reveals substantial discordance in magnitude and kinetics between inbred and outbred hosts. *J. Immunol.* **183,** 7672.

Rothe, J., Lesslauer, W., Lotscher, H., Lang, Y., Koebel, P., Kontgen, F., Althage, A., Zinkernagel, R., Steinmetz, M., and Bluethmann, H. (1993). Mice lacking the tumour necrosis factor receptor 1 are resistant to TNF-mediated toxicity but highly susceptible to infection by Listeria monocytogenes. *Nature* **364,** 798.

Sallusto, F., Lenig, D., Forster, R., Lipp, M., and Lanzavecchia, A. (1999). Two subsets of memory T lymphocytes with distinct homing potentials and effector functions. *Nature* **401,** 708.

San Mateo, L. R., Chua, M. M., Weiss, S. R., and Shen, H. (2002). Perforin-mediated CTL cytolysis counteracts direct cell-cell spread of Listeria monocytogenes. *J. Immunol.* **169,** 5202.

Sano, G., Hafalla, J. C., Morrot, A., Abe, R., Lafaille, J. J., and Zavala, F. (2001). Swift development of protective effector functions in naive CD8(+) T cells against malaria liver stages. *J. Exp. Med.* **194,** 173.

Schafer, R., Portnoy, D. A., Brassell, S. A., and Paterson, Y. (1992). Induction of a cellular immune response to a foreign antigen by a recombinant Listeria monocytogenes vaccine. *J. Immunol.* **149,** 53.

Schluns, K. S., and Lefrancois, L. (2003). Cytokine control of memory T-cell development and survival. *Nat. Rev. Immunol.* **3,** 269.

Schluns, K. S., Kieper, W. C., Jameson, S. C., and Lefrancois, L. (2000). Interleukin-7 mediates the homeostasis of naive and memory CD8 T cells in vivo. *Nat. Immunol.* **1,** 426.

Schmidt, N. W., Podyminogin, R. L., Butler, N. S., Badovinac, V. P., Tucker, B. J., Bahjat, K. S., Lauer, P., Reyes-Sandoval, A., Hutchings, C. L., Moore, A. C., Gilbert, S. C., Hill, A. V., *et al.* (2008). Memory CD8 T cell responses exceeding a large but definable threshold provide long-term immunity to malaria. *Proc. Natl. Acad. Sci. USA* **105,** 14017.

Schmidt, N. W., Butler, N. S., Badovinac, V. P., and Harty, J. T. (2010). Extreme CD8 T cell requirements for anti-malarial liver-stage immunity following immunization with radiation attenuated sporozoites. *PLoS Pathog.* **6,** e1000998.

Shen, H., Slifka, M. K., Matloubian, M., Jensen, E. R., Ahmed, R., and Miller, J. F. (1995). Recombinant Listeria monocytogenes as a live vaccine vehicle for the induction of protective anti-viral cell-mediated immunity. *Proc. Natl. Acad. Sci. USA* **92,** 3987.

Shen, H., Miller, J. F., Fan, X., Kolwyck, D., Ahmed, R., and Harty, J. T. (1998). Compartmentalization of bacterial antigens: Differential effects on priming of CD8 T cells and protective immunity. *Cell* **92,** 535.

Skoberne, M., and Geginat, G. (2002). Efficient in vivo presentation of Listeria monocytogenes- derived CD4 and CD8 T cell epitopes in the absence of IFN-gamma. *J. Immunol.* **168,** 1854.

Stavru, F., Archambaud, C., and Cossart, P. (2011). Cell biology and immunology of Listeria monocytogenes infections: Novel insights. *Immunol. Rev.* **240,** 160.

Sun, J. C., Williams, M. A., and Bevan, M. J. (2004). CD4+ T cells are required for the maintenance, not programming, of memory CD8+ T cells after acute infection. *Nat. Immunol.* **5,** 927.

Sun, J. C., Lehar, S. M., and Bevan, M. J. (2006). Augmented IL-7 signaling during viral infection drives greater expansion of effector T cells but does not enhance memory. *J. Immunol.* **177,** 4458.

Thompson, L. J., Kolumam, G. A., Thomas, S., and Murali-Krishna, K. (2006). Innate inflammatory signals induced by various pathogens differentially dictate the IFN-I dependence of CD8 T cells for clonal expansion and memory formation. *J. Immunol.* **177,** 1746.

van Stipdonk, M. J., Lemmens, E. E., and Schoenberger, S. P. (2001). Naive CTLs require a single brief period of antigenic stimulation for clonal expansion and differentiation. *Nat. Immunol.* **2,** 423.

Wherry, E. J., Teichgraber, V., Becker, T. C., Masopust, D., Kaech, S. M., Antia, R., von Andrian, U. H., and Ahmed, R. (2003). Lineage relationship and protective immunity of memory CD8 T cell subsets. *Nat. Immunol.* **4,** 225.

Wherry, E. J., Barber, D. L., Kaech, S. M., Blattman, J. N., and Ahmed, R. (2004). Antigen-independent memory CD8 T cells do not develop during chronic viral infection. *Proc. Natl. Acad. Sci. USA* **101,** 16004.

Wherry, E. J., Ha, S. J., Kaech, S. M., Haining, W. N., Sarkar, S., Kalia, V., Subramaniam, S., Blattman, J. N., Barber, D. L., and Ahmed, R. (2007). Molecular signature of CD8+ T cell exhaustion during chronic viral infection. *Immunity* **27,** 670.

Whitmire, J. K., Tan, J. T., and Whitton, J. L. (2005). Interferon-gamma acts directly on CD8+ T cells to increase their abundance during virus infection. *J. Exp. Med.* **201,** 1053.

Wing, E. J., and Gregory, S. H. (2000). From hot dogs to CD8+ T cells: Listeria monocytogenes. *Trans. Am. Clin. Climatol. Assoc.* **111,** 76.

Wirth, T. C., Xue, H. H., Rai, D., Sabel, J. T., Bair, T., Harty, J. T., and Badovinac, V. P. (2010). Repetitive antigen stimulation induces stepwise transcriptome diversification but preserves a core signature of memory CD8(+) T cell differentiation. *Immunity* **33,** 128.

Wong, P., and Pamer, E. G. (2001). Cutting edge: Antigen-independent CD8 T cell proliferation. *J. Immunol.* **166,** 5864.

Woodland, D. L. (2004). Jump-starting the immune system: Prime-boosting comes of age. *Trends Immunol.* **25,** 98.

Xiao, Z., Casey, K. A., Jameson, S. C., Curtsinger, J. M., and Mescher, M. F. (2009). Programming for CD8 T cell memory development requires IL-12 or type I IFN. *J. Immunol.* **182,** 2786.

Yewdell, J. W., and Bennink, J. R. (1999). Immunodominance in major histocompatibility complex class I-restricted T lymphocyte responses. *Annu. Rev. Immunol.* **17,** 51.

Zhao, X., Zhang, M., Li, Z., and Frankel, F. R. (2006). Vaginal protection and immunity after oral immunization of mice with a novel vaccine strain of Listeria monocytogenes expressing human immunodeficiency virus type 1 gag. *J. Virol.* **80,** 8880.

CHAPTER 6

Listeria monocytogenes and Its Products as Agents for Cancer Immunotherapy

Patrick Guirnalda,[1] **Laurence Wood,**[1] and **Yvonne Paterson**

Contents

Abstract

This review covers the use of *Listeria monocytogenes* and its virulence factors as cancer immunotherapeutics. We describe their development as vectors to carry protein tumor antigen and

Department of Microbiology, Perelman School of Medicine, University of Pennsylvania, Philadelphia, Pennsylvania, USA

[1] These authors contributed equally to this work.

Advances in Immunology, Volume 113
ISSN 0065-2776, DOI: 10.1016/B978-0-12-394590-7.00004-X

eukaryotic DNA plasmids to antigen-presenting cells and efforts to harness their tumor-homing properties. We also describe their use as vectors of angiogenic molecules to induce an immune response that will destroy tumor vasculature. The background knowledge necessary to understand the biology behind the rationale to develop *Listeria* as a vaccine vector for tumor immunotherapy is included as well as a brief summary of the major therapies that have used this approach thus far.

1. THE CHALLENGE OF TUMOR IMMUNOTHERAPY

The discovery of tumor-associated antigens (TAAs) three decades ago promoted the development of immunotherapy directed against them to eliminate cancer cells. These TAAs are often endogenous self-proteins (Van den Eynde *et al.*, 1989), which are either overexpressed or have unregulated expression. As most of these are located in the cytosol of the tumor cell, it is now believed that the most effective approach for tumor immunotherapy will require the induction of activated effector cytotoxic T lymphocytes (CTL) directed against TAAs, which can lyse and kill tumor cells. Thus, the latest cancer-vaccination strategies are primarily directed toward orchestrating strong antitumor-specific T cell responses by introducing identified T cell antigens to the immune system. The aim is to induce immune responses capable of eliminating primary and metastatic cancer. Since the majority of tumor antigens bear strong homology to self-proteins, they may have already been presented to the immune system in the context of tumor cells, which are poor antigen-presenting cells (APCs), under circumstances that induce peripheral tolerance. In addition, the chronic stimulation of the immune system by slow-growing tumors over years can also result in immunosuppression characterized by the presence of regulatory T cells and myeloid-derived suppressor cells (Drake *et al.*, 2006). Thus, the immune system of a tumor-bearing patient is likely to have undergone peripheral and/or central tolerance to TAAs rather than active T cell responses and to be in a state of immunosuppression. The challenge of tumor immunotherapy is to overcome these obstacles and "jump-start" the immune response to poor and/or tolerogenic tumor antigens.

One way of tackling this problem is to harness the proinflammatory properties of pathogens in order to overcome tolerance and enhance tumor antigenicity. Some pathogens that have been explored as vectors for tumor antigens are adenovirus, AAV, vaccinia, avipox, polio, VEEV, retrovirus, and the bacterial vectors *BCG*, *Escherichia coli*, *Chlamydia*, *Shigella*, *Salmonella*, *Listeria monocytogenes*, and *Streptococcus*. We believe that the biological properties of *Listeria* are particularly suited for this purpose since it shares with viruses the ability to locate antigens in the endogenous pathway of antigen presentation to cytotoxic T cells. In addition, it has advantages over viral vectors in that its infection can be easily terminated with antibiotics and the bacteria can be cheaply produced in simple media free from animal products and cells. Of course, the useful application of pathogens for human benefit necessitates the attenuation of their pathogenic properties, which can be achieved through deletion or alteration of their virulence factors.

Interestingly, the earliest form of cancer immunotherapy, which dates back to the nineteenth century, utilized bacteria. William Coley, a New York city surgeon in the 1880s, noted tumor regression in cancer patients after they contracted acute bacterial infections (Coley, 1893; McCarthy, 2006). He thus adopted the deliberate infection of patients with live bacteria (*Streptococcus*) as therapy for inoperable malignant cancer. Later, in collaboration with Robert Koch, he developed a mix of bacterial toxins for use in the treatment of cancer (Coley, 1909; McCarthy, 2006). Concerns regarding the efficacy and safety of ''Coley's toxins'' coupled with the development of chemo- and radiotherapy led to a decline in their use for cancer treatment by the middle of twentieth century. We can now identify many of the antitumor effector immune responses induced by bacteria, which include angiostatic effects induced by proinflammatory cytokines such as IL-12 and IFN-gamma, direct tumor necrosis by TNF-alpha, induction of epitope—spreading to TAAs induced by the death of tumor cells from these indirect mechanisms and the direct killing of tumor cells infected by bacteria. In this review, we discuss these mechanisms in the context of *L. monocytogenes* infection, in addition to its properties as a vector for presenting TAAs to the immune system.

2. THE BIOLOGY OF *L. MONOCYTOGENES*

Facultative intracellular bacteria, such as *Listeria*, are organisms that are free living but have evolved virulence factors that allow them to infect host animal cells and enable them to survive the microbicidal environment of phagocytic cells. Key to understanding the potential of intracellular bacteria as carriers of passenger antigens to the immune system is a knowledge of their cellular localization and mechanisms for inducing immunity, topics that will be covered in detail in other chapters of this volume. Bacterial products can signal through toll-like receptors and induce an inflammatory cytokine cascade that drives potent cellular immune responses against pathogens as well as tumors. The burst of innate immunity that precedes the adaptive immune response must be overcome for a successful infection to take place. In order to survive the microbicidal environment of the phagosome, intracellular bacteria secrete a variety of virulence factors that modify phagolysosomal microbicides such as defensins, reactive oxygen and nitrogen intermediates, and lysosomal enzymes that are active at acidic pH. Some mechanisms are common to many intracellular bacteria. Bacterial superoxide dismutase and catalase, for example, are common virulence factors, which act to neutralize the bactericidal activity of reactive oxygen intermediates. The exact mechanisms of many virulence genes are unknown, but there are indeed a large number that testify to the ingenuity of these bacteria in adapting to life inside the cell.

L. monocytogenes is unusual among the facultative intracellular bacteria because of its ability to escape the hostile environment of the phagolysosome and to colonize the cytosol of the host cell. *Listeriae* initially bind to host cells via surface proteins, such as internalins, and are phagocytosed (see Chapter 3). Once inside the phagosome, *Listeria* releases listeriolysin O (LLO) and phospholipase C (PLC), degrading the phagolysosome. *Listeriae* are then released into the cytoplasm where they multiply and become motile via the expression of ActA, a bacterial protein that enables actin mobilization. Motile bacteria then protrude out of the host cell and are subsequently phagocytosed by additional phagocytes in which they repeat the process (see Chapter 3). The intracellular localization of the bacterium necessitates cellular immune responses with a vital role for cytotoxic T cells in the clearance of infection. Indeed, *Listeria* is a well-studied model organism within the context of $CD8^+$ T cell responses (see Chapter 5).

The uptake of bacteria by phagocytic cells promotes not only changes in the microbicidal properties of the phagolysosomal compartment but also in the antigen-presenting function of these cells to the adaptive arm of the immune system. Bacterial phagocytosis stimulates macrophages to secrete a variety of humoral factors. These include chemokines that recruit new cells to the site of infection, inflammatory cytokines that increase vascular permeability, autocrines that promote the expression of MHC molecules and molecules associated with antigen processing, and lymphokines that act to promote cell-mediated immunity. A key lymphokine in this process is IL-12. Macrophages are stimulated by intracellular bacteria to release IL-12. This, in turn, promotes the production of IFN-gamma by NK cells, which has been shown to be a key factor in early host defense mechanisms against intracellular bacteria such as *Listeria* (Biron and Gazzinelli, 1995). In addition to its potent effects on innate immunity, IFN-gamma acts to direct the antigen-specific $CD4^+$ T cell response to the Th1 phenotype required to generate $CD8^+$ T cells and clear bacterial infection via adaptive cell-mediated immunity.

The cytokine-driven activation of macrophages that occurs early in infection will fail to kill *Listeriae* that have retreated into the cytoplasm of the cell. However, the presence of live bacteria in the cytosol facilitates the generation of $CD8^+$ CTL T cells that detect and lyse infected cells, which display antigenic peptides bound to MHC class I molecules. The generation of these peptides by the ubiquitin/proteosome pathway takes place in the cytosol of the cell after which they are transported to the endoplasmic reticulum by specialized chaperone molecules and loaded onto MHC class I molecules. Thus, bacterial virulence factors that are secreted by these bacteria into the cytosol become a potent source of peptides for the generation of CTL. $CD8^+$ cells are essential for the clearance of listerial infections and CTL have been found that are specific for many of the secreted listerial virulence factors that are required for phagosomal lysis and cell-to-cell spread (Pamer *et al.*, 1997). The ability of *Listeria* to target the MHC class I pathway of antigen processing has been a primary motive for the exploitation of these bacteria as vaccine vectors (Paterson *et al.*, 2010; Weiskirch and Paterson, 1997).

2.1. *L. monocytogenes* as a vaccine vector for cancer

The first paper to show that *Listeria* could target passenger antigens to the cellular arm of the immune system was published two decades ago. Since then *Listeria* has been viewed as an otherwise pathogenic organism that possesses potential therapeutic value as a vaccine vector. The intracellular lifestyle of *Listeria* ultimately leads to the activation of both $CD4^+$ and $CD8^+$ T cell-mediated adaptive immune responses as well as innate, proinflammatory cytokine responses (see Chapter 5). The first attempt to use *Listeria* as a vector to target antigens to the immune system was published by our laboratory in 1992 (Schafer *et al.*, 1992). Although this paper demonstrated that a $CD8^+$ T cell response to a passenger antigen could be induced by *Listeria*, its utility in cancer was not established until 1995, when we showed that *Listeria* expressing and secreting a tumor-specific antigen could control tumor growth largely mediated by a $CD8^+$ T cell mechanism (Pan *et al.*, 1995a). In this study, we used the influenza antigen, nucleoprotein (NP) as a model antigen to test the ability of *Listeria* expressing NP (Lm-NP) to protect against challenge by NP expressing tumor lines and to eradicate established tumors from several different tissues (Pan *et al.*, 1995a,b, 1999). We used an expression system in which the NP antigen was expressed as a fusion protein consisting of a truncated and nonfunctional virulence factor, LLO, joined to the NP. To ensure retention of the plasmid *in vivo*, a copy of the *prfA* gene was included on the plasmid, which was then used to transform a *prfA*-negative mutant of *L. monocytogenes* that is incapable of *in vivo* replication in the absence of the episomal expression of *prfA* (Ikonomidis *et al.*, 1994).

To test the ability of Lm-NP to act as a tumor immunotherapeutic, we used the transplantable BALB/c mouse-derived tumors CT26-NP and Renca-NP (Pan *et al.*, 1995a). Not only did Lm-NP treatment protect mice in a NP-specific manner from subsequent tumor challenge, but it also induced the complete regression of established tumors. This study also verified the importance of $CD8^+$ T cells to the efficacy of the Lm-NP vaccine in that not only did Lm-NP immunization induce CTLs that lysed CT26-NP and Renca-NP *in vitro* but also depletion of $CD8^+$ T cells *in vivo* completely abrogated the antitumor efficacy of Lm-NP. $CD4^+$ T cells were also shown to be important for protection from tumor challenge since Lm-NP immunized mice that were depleted of $CD4^+$ T cells prior to tumor challenge were only able to slow the growth of the CT26-NP tumors, not to reject them. Importantly, this was the first paper to show that an induced immune response against a TAA could eliminate established tumors without other adjunctive therapy (Pan *et al.*, 1995a). This groundbreaking experiment is shown in Fig. 6.1. Since then, a number of investigators have used *Listeria* to target many different TAAs (Paterson *et al.*, 2010; Wallecha *et al.*, 2009a) and a complete list is shown in Table 6.1. They include both natural tumor antigens such as PSA, Mage-b, HER-2/neu, p53, TRP-2, and HPV-16 E7 as well as the use of viral proteins, such as influenza and LCMV NPs as model tumor antigen targets. These recombinant, protein-expressing strains of *Listeria* have been tested in mouse models of melanoma, prostate, breast, cervical, renal, and colon cancer. In this review, we focus on our own studies, including more recent studies that concentrated on overcoming a variety of physiological barriers against efficacious immunotherapeutic treatments of cancer. Specifically, protein products produced and secreted by the bacterium, such as LLO and ActA, have been fused to tumor antigens in order to increase the antigenicity of otherwise poorly immunogenic tumor antigens in animal models of cancer.

The primary cellular targets for *Listeria* are phagocytic cells; however, *Listeria* can also infect epithelial cells, and recent reports show that *Listeria* can also infect tumor cells directly (Huang *et al.*, 2007; Kim *et al.*, 2009). The ability of *Listeria* to infect phagocytic cells, including APCs such as macrophages and DCs, is of particular interest since *Listeria* engineered to express TAAs could prime or reactivate tumor-specific T cells that are capable of killing tumors. After phagocytosis by an APC, *Listeria* escapes the phagosome via the hemolytic virulence factor LLO and enters the cytoplasm. In our laboratory, we engineered *Listeria* to express our genes of interest under the LLO (*hly*) promoter. In addition to delivering our antigen in a bacterial vector that will drive strong inflammatory responses, we fuse our gene of interest to the virulence factors LLO or ActA. In general, tumors are poorly immunogenic; however, studies in our lab and others have shown that *Listeria* is a particularly good vector for TAA immunization (Gunn *et al.*, 2001; Seavey *et al.*, 2008; Sewell *et al.*, 2004a,b; Shahabi *et al.*, 2008; Singh *et al.*, 2005).

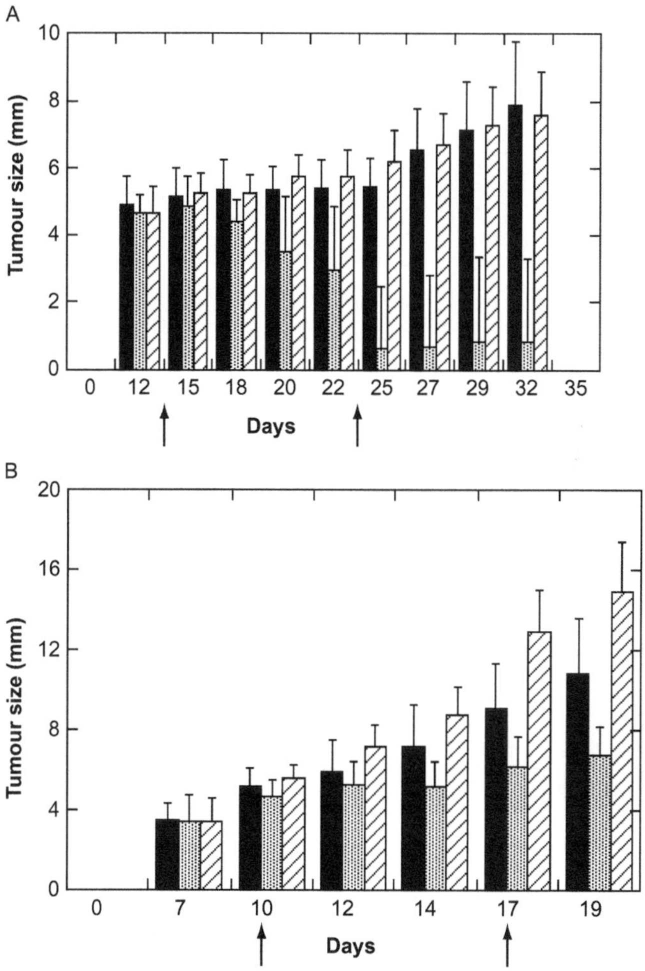

FIGURE 6.1 The first demonstration of the elimination of established tumors in mice by a *Listeria*-based immunotherapy. The tumor cell lines Renca (a renal carcinoma) and CT26 (a colorectal carcinoma), which had been transduced with influenza nucleoprotein (NP), were established in syngeneic mice. 5×10^5 tumor cells of either Renca-NP (A) or CT26-NP (B) were introduced subcutaneously to two groups of 30 mice. After measurable tumors had grown in the mice, in each group, 10 mice received a *Listeria monocytogenes* (Lm) recombinant that expressed and secreted NP fused to a truncated form of LLO, Lm-NP (darkly shaded bars), 10 mice received wild-type *Listeria* (lightly shaded bars), and 10 received saline (solid bars). The mice received immunizations on the days indicated by the arrows. Reprinted by permission from McMillan Publishers Ltd.: Pan *et al.*, 1995a, copyright 1995.

TABLE 6.1 Live *Listeria*-based tumor antigen delivery systems tested *in vivo* in animal models of cancer; this table only includes those studies where the antigen is delivered as a *Listeria* expressed and secreted protein

Antigen	Cancer model	Origin of antigen	Vaccine name	Host strain	Expression system	References
E7	Cervical	HPV-16	Lm-LLO-E7	*prfA*–	Plasmid	Gunn *et al.* (2001)
			Lm-E7	wild-type	Chromosomal	Gunn *et al.* (2001)
			Lm-PEST-E7	*prfA*–	Plasmid	Sewell *et al.* (2004b)
			Lm-ActA-E7	*prfA*–	Plasmid	Sewell *et al.* (2004a)
			rLm-E7	wild-type	Chromosomal	Lin *et al.* (2002)
			Lm-dd-LLO-E7	dal–, dat–	Plasmid	Verch *et al.* (2004)
L1	Cervical	HPV-16	Lm-LLO-L1(1–258)	*prfA*–	Plasmid	Mustafa *et al.* (2009)
E1	Papilloma	CRPV	Lm-LLO-L1(238–474)	*prfA*–	Plasmid	Mustafa *et al.* (2009)
			E1-rLM	wild-type	Chromosomal	Jensen *et al.* (1997)
Her2/neu	Breast	Rat	Lm-LLO-EC1	*prfA*–	Plasmid	Singh *et al.* (2005)
		Human	Lm-LLO-EC2	*prfA*–	Plasmid	Singh *et al.* (2005)
			Lm-LLO-EC3	*prfA*–	Plasmid	Singh *et al.* (2005)
			Lm-LLO-IC1	*prfA*–	Plasmid	Singh *et al.* (2005)
			Lm-LLO-IC2	*prfA*–	Plasmid	Singh *et al.* (2005)
			Lm-LLO-chHer-2/neu (chimera)	*prfA*–	Plasmid	Seavey *et al.* (2009a)
			Lm-LLO-chHer-2/neu*ddA* (chimera)	*dal* –, *dat* –, *actA* –	Plasmid	Shahabi *et al.* (2011)
Flk-1 (VEGFR2)	Breast	Mouse	Lm-LLO-Flk-E1	*prfA*–	Plasmid	Seavey *et al.* (2009b)
			Lm-LLO-Flk-E2	*prfA*–	Plasmid	Seavey *et al.* (2009b)
			Lm-LLO-Flk-I1	*prfA*–	Plasmid	Seavey *et al.* (2009b)

Endoglin (CD105)	Breast	Mouse	Lm-LLO-CD105A	*prfA*−	Plasmid	Wood *et al*. (2011a)
			Lm-LLO-CD105B	*prfA*−	Plasmid	Wood *et al*. (2011a)
MAGE-b3	Breast	Mouse	Lm-LLO-Mage-b311-660	*prfA*−	Plasmid	Kim *et al*. (2008)
ISG15	Breast	Mouse	Lm-LLO-ISG15	*prfA*−	Plasmid	Wood *et al*. (2011b)
p53	Breast	Human	Lm-ddA-LLO-p53	*dal*−, *dat*−, *actA*−	Plasmid	Ishizaki *et al*. (2010)
TRP-2	Melanoma	Mouse	Lm-TRP2	wild-type	Chromosomal	Bruhn *et al*. (2005)
HMW-MAA		Human	Lm-LLO–HMW-MAA-C	*prfA*−	Plasmid	Maciag *et al*. (2008)
GP70, AH1 epitope	Colon	MuLV	actA-inlb-Ah1-A5	actA−, inlb−	Chromosomal by phage integration	Brockstedt *et al*. (2004)
PSA	Prostate	Human	Lm-LLO-PSA	*prfA*−	Plasmid	Shahabi *et al*. (2008)
			Lm-dal dat actA 142	*dal*−, *dat*−, *actA*−	Plasmid	Wallecha *et al*. (2009b)
Nucleoprotein (NP)	Colon, renal Melanoma	Influenza	Lm-NP	*prfA*−	Plasmid	Pan *et al*. (1995a,b) Pan *et al*. (1999)
Nucleoprotein (NP)	CNS	LCMV	rLm-NP	wild-type	Chromosomal	Liau *et al*. (2002)
E. coli beta-galactosidase	Fibrosarcoma	*E. coli*	Dmpl2GK20	*Delta mpl2*	Plasmid	Paglia *et al*. (1997)

2.2. *Listeria* targeting HPV-16 E7 as a vaccine for cervical cancer

Human papilloma viruses (HPVs) are a heterogeneous group of viruses with over 100 different subtypes that inhabit the squamous epithelium of the mucocutaneous surface. Acute infections cause either minor subclinical disease or chronic infections characterized by the formation of papillomas. Severe life-threatening disease occurs when chronic infection, caused by a small subset of about 14 serotypes of papilloma viruses, leads to malignant disease (Tindle, 1996). Although the immune system is effective in eliminating HPV-infected cells in most healthy people, HPV can establish a chronic infection in a significant percentage of women, which can lead to cervical cancer when the papilloma infection involves malignant serotypes. Thus, there is a need to change the immune response in individuals with inadequate immune responses to HPV, either qualitatively or quantitatively, so as to treat chronic HPV infections and associated neoplastic disease. This requires the development of an effective cytotoxic T cell response against viral antigens expressed during the chronic phase of infection or after transformation of host cells has taken place.

Cervical cancer is the second most common female malignancy, inducing disease in over 400,000 women per year worldwide and is a leading cause of death when not detected early. HPV serotypes 16 and 18 are the primary cause of anogentital cancer and are strongly associated with certain forms of head and neck cancer. Both cervical and squamous cell carcinomas of the tonsil show correlation with HPV-16 (Gillison *et al.*, 2000; Lowy *et al.*, 1994). HPV encodes three transforming oncogenes: E5, E6, and E7. The early transforming proteins, E6 and E7, are almost ideal candidates for vaccine approaches against HPV neoplasia because they are constitutively expressed in HPV-transformed tissues and are thought to be necessary to maintain the transformed state of these cells (Seedorf *et al.*, 1987). In addition, there is a wealth of evidence that these two proteins are immunogenic in humans with the production of both humoral- and cell-mediated responses (Tindle and Frazer, 1994). Both E6 and E7 are responsible for the induction of cancer by binding to and inhibiting the function of two major tumor suppressor proteins, p53 and pRb respectively (Scheffner *et al.*, 1990), which play major roles in cellular replication and DNA damage/repair. Thus, the actions of E6 and E7 in the cervix epithelium lead to epithelial cells becoming immortalized, which ultimately leads to neoplasia and cervical cancer.

To test *Listeria*-based therapeutics for cervical cancer, we have used two mouse models for HPV-induced cancer. One requires transplanting tumors subcutaneously in the normal mouse and the other measures the spontaneous growth of tumors in a transgenic mouse model. For the experiments using transplantable tumors, we employed the HPV-16 E6 and E7 immortalized mouse tumor line TC-1 to test the antitumor effectiveness of the E7-specific immune responses induced by E7 secreting *Listeria* strains. TC-1 is a lung epithelial cell immortalized by HPV-16 E6 and E7 and transformed by pVEJB-expressing activated human c-Ha-*ras* (Lin *et al.*, 1996). It is an aggressive tumor, syngeneic with the C57Bl/6 mouse. Like human HPV-associated tumors, TC-1 constitutively expresses E6 and E7. We constructed two *Listeria* strains that either secreted E7 alone or as a fusion protein consisting of a truncated LLO joined at the C-terminus to E7 (Gunn *et al.*, 2001). E7 is a small protein (98 residues) and was readily expressed and secreted by both *L. monocytogenes* recombinants. However, they induced very different antitumor therapeutic outcomes. Lm-LLO-E7 treatment effectively eradicated established TC-1 in the majority of tumor-bearing mice. *In vivo* antibody depletion studies demonstrated that the antitumor response required $CD4^+$ and $CD8^+$ T cells as well as IFN-gamma. However, Lm-E7 treatment of tumor-bearing mice had little impact on the growth of the tumor. Unexpectedly, the depletion of $CD4^+$ T cells greatly improved the effectiveness of the Lm-E7 treatment and induced the regression of TC-1 in about 25% of treated mice. This suggested that $CD4^+$ T cells induced by Lm-E7 were immunosuppressive. To test this hypothesis, we adoptively transferred $CD4^+$ T cells from mice immunized with Lm-E7 or a control *Listeria* vector. We found that $CD4^+$ T cells induced by Lm-E7, but not the control vector, which expressed an irrelevant antigen fused to LLO, could negate the anti-TC-1 immune response induced by Lm-LLO-E7-treated recipient mice (Gunn *et al.*, 2001).

We next determined whether the Lm-E7-induced immunosuppression was mediated by the $CD4^+CD25^+$ regulatory T cell subset (Tregs) important for the maintenance of self-tolerance (Sakaguchi *et al.*, 1995) and which have been shown to suppress both proliferation and IFN-gamma production by $CD8^+$ T cells (Piccirillo and Shevach, 2001). $CD4^+CD25^+$ Treg cells have also been demonstrated to aid tumor growth by suppressing antitumor immune responses (Onizuka *et al.*, 1999). Further, transforming growth factor-β (TGF-β) has been reported to be secreted by Treg cells (Read *et al.*, 2000) and to protect tumors from immune responses in immune competent hosts. (Chang *et al.*, 1993; Torre-Amione *et al.*, 1990) The depletion of both $CD25^+$ cells and TGF-β in Lm-E7-treated mice greatly improved the antitumor response (Gunn *et al.*, 2001). Further, we were able to demonstrate the presence of $CD4^+CD25^+$ T cells in the tumors of Lm-E7-immunized mice that secreted both TGF-β and IL-10 (Hussain and Paterson, 2004). Taken together, these studies demonstrate that recombinant listerial vectors have the potential to induce both effective and suppressive immunity.

In addition to the *Listeria*-based vaccine, Lm-LLO-E7, we have also created a recombinant *Listeria* that expresses E7 as a fusion protein with the virulence factor ActA, Lm-ActA-E7, as an alternative vaccine for HPV-16-induced cancers (Sewell *et al.*, 2004a). As we did for LLO, we truncated the ActA virulence factor to remove possible cell cytotoxicity. Our reason for using ActA as a fusion protein was because it also contains PEST sequences. LLO contains an N-terminal PEST sequence, which is a region rich in the following amino acids: proline (P), glutamic acid (E), serine (S), threonine (T) (Sewell *et al.*, 2004b). This region is thought to regulate intracellular levels of LLO after *Listeria* has entered the cytosol (Decatur and Portnoy, 2000). At first, it was suggested that the PEST region rapidly targeted the LLO protein for host degradation by the ubiquitin–proteosome pathway (Decatur and Portnoy, 2000), but this explanation has now been called into question and it is thought instead to be involved in modulating translation of mRNA (Schnupf *et al.*, 2006). Nonetheless, we have found that including the PEST region of LLO, and similar sequences in ActA, conveys adjuvant properties and significantly enhanced the immunogenicity of the fused antigen (Gunn *et al.*, 2001; Sewell *et al.*, 2004a,b). Both Lm-LLO-E7 and Lm-ActA-E7 vaccines induce CTLs that can penetrate and kill the solid tumor in the transplantable TC-1 tumor model syngeneic with C57Bl/6 mice (Gunn *et al.*, 2001; Hussain and Paterson, 2005; Sewell *et al.*, 2004a,b).

A major problem with using transplantable tumors to test cancer immunotherapeutics is that they poorly mimic the growth of tumors in the human host, which may take decades and induce immune tolerance and immunosuppression, before presenting for treatment. We thus generated a mouse transgenic for HPV-16 E6 and E7 under the thyroglobulin promoter, which develops tumors around 6 months of age (Souders *et al.*, 2007). The genetic background of the E6/E7 transgenic mouse is identical to C57BL/6 except for the tissue-specific expression of the E6/E7 transgenes. E7 was expressed in these mice in the thyroid and in mouse thymic epithelial cells (mTECs), which are thought to present self-antigens to T cells in the thymus to ensure negative selection of high-avidity T cells responsive to tissue-specific antigens (Derbinski *et al.*, 2001). mTECs can delete autoreactive T cells either directly or indirectly by thymic dendritic cell (DC) cross-presentation of the peripheral antigen to the autoreactive T cell (Gallegos and Bevan, 2004). mTECs uniquely express the autoimmune regulator (AIRE) gene, which is a transcription factor critical for maintaining T cell tolerance to self-proteins (Anderson *et al.*, 2002; Liston *et al.*, 2003). AIRE controls the expression of peripheral antigens and their processing and presentation of those antigens (Anderson *et al.*, 2005). Mice in which the AIRE gene has been deleted rapidly succumb to a variety of autoimmune disorders directed toward peripheral tissue including the thyroid. mTECs thus play a critical role in deleting T cells reactive to thyroid antigens during repertoire selection in the thymus in an AIRE-dependent manner (Liston *et al.*, 2004). We thus predicted that these mice would be immune tolerant to E7 and found that the E7-specific $CD8^+$ T cell response induced by the *Listeria* vaccines, Lm-LLO-E7 and Lm-ActA-E7, were of lower avidity in the E6/E7 transgenic mouse compared to the wild-type mouse consistent with the expression of the E7 transgene in mTECs.

The expansion of E7-specific T cells in the transgenic mouse is probably due to the activation of low-avidity T cells that are not deleted during thymic selection. However, Lm-LLO-E7 and Lm-ActA-E7 still showed therapeutic efficacy in the E6/E7 transgenic mouse as measured by the eradication of implanted TC-1 tumors, although the wild-type mice mounted a more robust immune response presumably due to a lack of tolerance to the E7 antigen, allowing for a high-avidity anti-E7 CTL response (Souders *et al.*, 2007). More importantly, we could also show that both Lm-LLO-E7 and Lm-ActA-E7 can impact on the growth of autochthonous tumors that arise in the E6/E7 transgenic mouse in that early treatment with *Listeria* vaccines expressing E7 significantly reduced their thyroid tumors compared with mice treated with controls (Sewell *et al.*, 2008; see Fig. 6.2). In addition, higher numbers of antigen-specific $CD8^+$ T cells were found in the spleens, tumors, and peripheral blood in Lm-LLO-E7 and Lm-ActA-E7 vaccinated transgenic mice. This study shows that *Listeria*-based vaccines perform well in the more stringent model of autochthonous tumor growth.

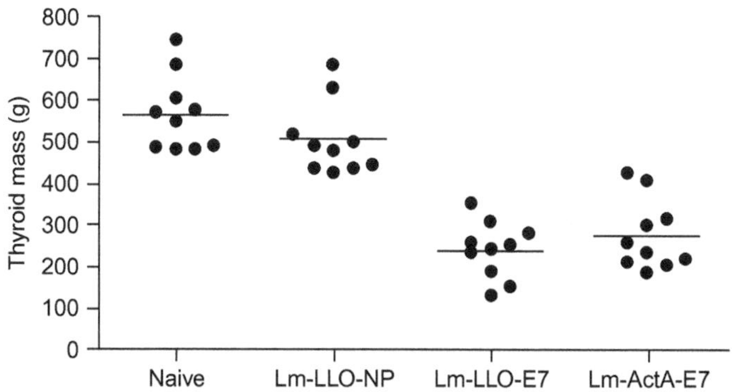

FIGURE 6.2 *Listeria*-based vaccines can overcome tolerance and control autochthonous tumor growth in E6/E7 transgenic mice. Six- to eight-week-old E6/E7 transgenic mice were divided into groups of 10 or 12 mice which were then immunized intraperitoneally (i.p.) with 0.1 LD_{50} Lm-LLO-E7, Lm-ActA-E7, Lm-LLO-NP, or left naive. The mice were immunized monthly for 8 months. At the end of 8 months, the thyroid tumors were excised and weighed. Individual sizes from each of the four groups are shown. The difference in average sizes between each of the experimental groups (Lm-ActA-E7 and Lm-LLO-E7) and the negative control groups (naïve and Lm-LLO-NP) is statistically significant ($P < 0.001$, one-way ANOVA) (Sewell *et al.*, 2008, pp. 5322–5327). Reprinted by permission from Elsevier, copyright 2008.

2.3. *Listeria*-based immunotherapy for breast cancer

About 15–40% of all breast carcinomas overexpress the epidermal-like growth factor HER-2/neu. Thus, this protein can act as a TAA and as a target for immunotherapy (Ercolini *et al.*, 2003; Seavey *et al.*, 2009a; Singh and Paterson 2006, 2007; Singh *et al.*, 2005). Since HER-2/neu is a large transmembrane molecule of >1200 residues, we initially targeted HER-2/neu by constructing five different *Listeria*-based constructs each expressing a different fragment of the HER-2/neu molecule, three fragments spanned the extracellular domain and two fragments covered the intracellular domain (Singh *et al.*, 2005). Since *Listeria* has difficulty in secreting hydrophobic regions, the transmembrane region and leader sequence were omitted. Each of the five *Listeria* constructs was able to impact tumor growth in a subcutaneous implanted mouse tumor model for breast cancer (Singh *et al.*, 2005). The use of *Listeria* as a shuttle vector revealed several CTL epitopes not previously identified (Singh and Paterson, 2006; Singh *et al.*, 2005) using killed tumor vaccines, vaccinia-based vaccines (Ercolini *et al.*, 2003), or DNA vaccines (Singh and Paterson, 2006). Indeed, our studies suggest that epitope immunodominance depends largely on the vaccination strategy in that fusion of the HER-2/neu antigen to LLO in a DNA vaccine increased the immune response to some epitopes and delivering the fusion antigen by *Listeria* further identified a number of epitope specificities in the immune response (Singh and Paterson, 2006).

We have extensively tested all of our *Listeria*-based HER-2/neu vaccines for their ability to impact on autochthonous tumors that arise in a mouse transgenic for rat HER-2/neu expressed from an MMTV promoter (Singh and Paterson, 2007). Female transgenic mice begin to develop breast tumors around 5 months of age, and by about 9 months, all female mice have tumors. By vaccinating mice at 6, 9, 12, 15, and 18 weeks of age, we could delay the onset of tumor growth by about 5 months using the *Listeria* vaccine that expressed a fragment of the intracellular domain that encompasses the tyrosine kinase domain of the molecule. Other HER-2/neu fragments were less successful at providing protection and eventually tumors did emerge in all vaccinated mice. To determine why the vaccines could only delay and not prevent tumor growth, we sequenced the HER-2/neu molecule expressed by the tumors that escaped and discovered that a number of mutations had arisen but only in the regions of the HER-2/neu molecule targeted by the *Listeria* strain expressing that region (see Table 6.2). This suggests that immunoediting of the HER-2/neu antigen occurred in response to immune pressure and that the rates of generation of escape mutants were a significant factor in the efficacy of each vaccine. The long delay in the onset of tumors after targeting the kinase domain we found was associated with the mutation of specific

TABLE 6.2 Productive mutations accumulate in regions of the HER-2/neu molecule that each vaccine targets a summary of data reported in Singh and Paterson (2007)

Vaccine used	Number of mutations in region EC1	Number of mutations in region EC2	Number of mutations in region EC3	Number of mutations in region IC1	Number of mutations in region IC2
Saline	1	0	2	0	1
Saline	1	1	0	0	2
Control Lm	1	2	1	1	1
Control Lm	1	0	1	1	1
Lm-EC1	5	1	0	0	0
Lm-EC1	5	0	1	2	1
Lm-EC2	1	5	0	1	2
Lm-EC2	1	6	0	1	1
Lm-EC3	2	1	5	1	1
Lm-EC3	1	0	6	1	0
Lm-IC1	1	2	0	7	0
Lm-IC1	0	1	1	7	1
Lm-IC2	1	0	2	1	14
Lm-IC2	1	0	0	0	9

residues outside the catalytic domain but which may be present in the ATP-binding domain. These mutations could alter the catalysis of ATP, which in turn could diminish signaling through the kinase domain and delay the growth of the tumors (Singh and Paterson, 2007). Thus, the enhanced success of the *Listeria* that expressed the tyrosine kinase region of HER-2/neu may be due to deleterious functional consequences of escape mutations.

In order to spread the immune pressure to mutate over a wider region of the HER-2/neu molecule, a *Listeria* strain was constructed that secretes a chimeric product composed of three immunodominant regions of three HER-2/neu fragments (Seavey *et al.*, 2009a). Vaccination with the HER-2/neu chimeric *Listeria* vaccine induced regression of established tumors and prevented lung metastasis in transplantable mouse models of breast cancer (Seavey *et al.*, 2009a). To further improve this vector for human use, the LLO-chimeric HER-2/neu fusion was introduced into a *Listeria* host strain that lacked *actA* (to improve safety) and also two genes that encode alanine racemases (*dal* and *dat*). This strain cannot grow *in vivo* or *in vitro* in the absence of D-alanine or unless a copy of an alanine racemase is included on the plasmid to complement this activity. This new complementation system, which was developed in our laboratory (Verch *et al.*, 2004), removes the need to include an antibiotic resistance gene to select for plasmid transformants since these can now be selected by growth in the absence of D-alanine. The chimeric HER-2/neu-LLO fusion vaccine delivered by this safer strain was as effective at eradicating established HER-2/neu expressing tumors in transplantable tumor models of breast cancer and more effective in preventing autochthonous tumor growth in the HER-2/neu transgenic mouse. This better therapeutic outcome correlated with reduced accumulation of mutations in tumors that grew out in vaccinated animals (Shahabi *et al.*, 2011).

3. THE PLEIOTROPIC EFFECTS OF *LISTERIA* IN TUMOR IMMUNOTHERAPY

When we first proposed using *L. monocytogenes* as a vaccine vector for TAAs, it was predicated on the ability of the pathogen to induce strong cell-mediated immunity (Pan *et al.*, 1995a). Indeed, $CD8^+$ T cells have been shown in all of our studies to be the key effector cell in eliminating tumors. However, the induction of CTL, although a necessary condition for effective immunotherapy, is not a sufficient condition (Hussain and Paterson, 2005). Effector $CD4^+$ T cells, APCs, and an array of cytokines and chemokines also play a role in tumor regression. Vaccination with *Listeria* vaccines not only induces $CD8^+$ CTLs but also initiates a standard sequence of events that involves the sequential or coordinated activation and movement of innate and adaptive cells.

Using a variety of vectors designed to induce strong CTL responses against HPV-16 and eliminate the TC-1 tumor in mice, we have shown a near perfect correlation with eradication of established tumors and the presence of IFN-gamma secreting anti-E7 CTL in the tumor ($R = 0.9$) whereas a less robust correlation exists between tumor eradication and their induction in the spleen ($R = 0.3$) (Hussain and Paterson 2005). Clearly, the induced $CD8^+$ T cells must be able to home to and penetrate the tumor, and the best vaccine vectors such as Lm-LLO-E7 and Lm-ActA-E7 induce additional responses to facilitate appropriate immune cell trafficking. Proinflammatory cytokines, particularly IFN-gamma, are necessary for vaccine-mediated tumor regression (Gunn *et al.*, 2001). IFN-gamma, secreted early in the innate immune response to *Listeria* by NK cells and then later in the adaptive immune response by $CD4^+$ and $CD8^+$ T cells, plays a key role in mediating T cell infiltration into tumors. Antibody ablation of IFN-gamma in tumor-bearing mice inhibited vaccine-mediated regression (Gunn *et al.*, 2001). Subsequent studies showed that genetically altered implanted TC-1 tumors that overexpress a dominant/negative IFN-gamma receptor failed to regress on vaccination with Lm-LLO-E7 and that $CD8^+$ T cells failed to infiltrate the tumor matrix (Dominiecki *et al.*, 2005). T cell homing and infiltration is typically governed by chemokines that are regulated by a variety of proinflammatory cytokines. Recently, we have shown that TC-1 and a wide variety of other mouse tumors respond to IFN-gamma by expressing a variety of chemokines including the CXCL cytokines 9 and 10 (Guirnalda *et al.*, in preparation). Interestingly, over half of the E7-specific $CD8^+$ tumor infiltrating T cells found in TC-1 tumors after vaccination with Lm-LLO-E7 express CXCR3, the receptor for these ligands. Antigen-specific effector $CD8^+$ T cells have been shown to upregulate CXCR3 during the course of infection (Hu *et al.*, 2011), and CXCR3 T cell tumor infiltration generally correlates with tumor regression or positive prognosis in a variety of cancers and cancer models. In addition to its ability to promote chemokine-directed T cell infiltration, IFN-gamma can also inhibit angiogenesis at the tumor site in the early effector phase following vaccination (Beatty and Paterson, 2001) either directly or through the generation of angiostatic CXCR3 ligands.

The ability of *Listeria* to induce strong cell-mediated immunity, characterized by Th1 and CTL cells, is related to its propensity to infect and mature DCs. On infection of DCs, *Listeria* induces the release of IL-2, IL-6, IL-12, and TNF-alpha from DCs and also upregulates cell surface expression of costimulatory molecules CD40, B7-H1 (PD-L1), CD86 (B7-2), and B7-DC (PD-L2) that results in the maturation and activation of high-affinity T cells (Peng *et al.*, 2004). The production of IL-12, IL-6, and TNF-alpha is most efficiently triggered by cytosolic *Listeria*, and LLO is required for optimal T cell priming and cytokine production that result in functionally therapeutic CTL responses (Brzoza *et al.*, 2004). In humans, *Listeria* infection also results in the maturation of DCs that display high levels of CD83, CD25, MHC Class II, and CD86 (Kolb-Mäurer *et al.*, 2000). Kinetic studies in mice have shown that infection with *Listeria* results in a tissue-specific expansion of conventional DC (cDC) and plasmacytoid DC (pDC) followed by an upregulation of CD80 and CD86 on cDC, which are an important source of IL-12, in spleen and mesenteric lymph nodes. Expansion of pDC is more prolonged than cDC (Tam and Wick, 2006).

A major challenge in applying a T cell based cancer immunotherapy is the presence of $FoxP3^+$ regulatory T cells in the tumor. Frequently, tumors have evolved to exploit the suppressive properties of these regulatory cells in order to promote their growth and persistence within the host. The presence of Tregs can suppress therapeutic T cell responses and some immunotherapies can actually induce Tregs (Gunn *et al.*, 2001). However, Lm-LLO based vaccines, which express antigen-LLO fusion proteins, appear to proportionally reduce Tregs in established tumors. For example, immunization with Lm-LLO-E7 fusion protein resulted in fewer Tregs ($CD4^+$, $CD25^+$ cells) in the tumors when compared to Lm-E7 that secretes the antigen, but not the LLO-antigen fusion protein (Hussain and Paterson, 2004). Interestingly, immunization with a nonspecific *Listeria* expressing an LLO-irrelevant antigen vaccine also results in a reduced percentage of Tregs within tumors (Shahabi *et al.*, 2008), although this reduction is not as profound as when the vaccine was antigen specific, suggesting that the mechanism is at least partially antigen dependent for a maximal effect (Nitcheu-Tefit *et al.*, 2007; Shahabi *et al.*, 2008). A change in the proportions of Tregs in the tumors is not due to a significant decrease in the number found in the periphery such as the spleen (Hussain and Paterson, 2004). Rather, we think that the smaller percentage of $CD4^+$ $FoxP3^+$ T cells in the tumor is due to a large influx of $CD4^+$ $FoxP3^-$ Th1 cells present in the tumor, which may act to neutralize the immunosuppressive effects of the Tregs on effector $CD8^+$ T cells (P. Guirnalda and Y. Paterson, unpublished). Indeed, *Listeria* vaccines not only generate tumor antigen-specific $CD8^+$ T cells but also generate *Listeria*-specific cells including LLO-responsive $CD4^+$ T cells that likely provide necessary Th cytokines for maximal CD8 T cell responses (P. Guirnalda and Y. Paterson, unpublished). In the years since our initial characterizations of vaccine responses, we have learned that *Listeria* vaccines not only generate necessary $CD8^+$ T cells but also effectively coordinate the establishment of increased effector to regulatory T cell ratios in the tumor through a combination of cytokine, chemokine, and cellular responses.

Why some of our vaccines are more effective at creating a favorable proinflammatory environment and inducing critical subsets of tumor and bacterial-vector antigen specific T cells is under investigation; however, the interplay among antigen quality and construction, presentation and recognition, TCR specificity, and effector chemokine receptor expression, coupled with the ability of our bacterial vaccines to induce innate and adaptive cells to produce proinflammatory cytokines appears to be important in effecting key alterations within the tumor microenvironment to favor immune cell-mediated eradication.

4. THE USE OF *LISTERIA* TO TARGET TUMOR VASCULATURE

Because of the instability of tumor cells and tumor antigen expression, we sought a new tumor target that may be less susceptible to genetic mutation. Folkman and colleagues first suggested that tumor growth could be inhibited by attacking the tumor's vascular network (Folkman, 1971, 1996). Blood vessels, in general, are composed of two different cell types, the endothelial cells that line blood vessels and interact directly with the blood stream, and the pericytes, a cell type responsible for maintaining vascular integrity, which is found on the capillary cell wall. Both cell types are crucial to vascular function. Thus, we sought to determine whether *Listeria*-based vaccines could target molecules expressed by pericytes (Maciag *et al.*, 2008) or endothelial cells (Seavey *et al.*, 2009b; Wood *et al.*, 2011a).

One of the most important molecules in the formation of new blood vessels is the vascular endothelial growth factor receptor 2 (VEGFR2), which is called fetal liver kinase 1 (Flk-1) in the mouse. When tumors cells first begin to grow and divide, they can extract oxygen and nutrients from the interstitial fluid via passive diffusion, but once the tumor has reached a critical mass, 2–3 mm in diameter, the formation of new blood vessels is required. Thus, VEGFR2 is strongly indicated as a therapeutic target (Luo *et al.*, 2007; Niethammer *et al.*, 2002) to inhibit tumor growth, invasion, and metastasis (Shibuya, 2006).

Immunotherapeutic strategies that harness bacteria as a delivery mechanism for proangiogenic factors were first suggested by Reisfeld and colleagues who used DNA vaccines delivered orally by *Salmonella typhimurium* (Niethammer *et al.*, 2002). To construct *Listeria* vectors, we selected three polypeptide fragments of the VEGFR2 molecule and fused each to LLO (Seavey *et al.*, 2009b). The FLK-1 expressing *Listeria* vaccines were able to cause tumor regression, HER-2/neu epitope spreading, reduce tumor microvascular density (MVD), and prevent the long-term growth of spontaneous tumors all without significantly affecting normal tissue angiogenesis. In addition, tumors that escaped immune surveillance had acquired mutations in key regions of the HER-2/neu molecule responsible for both its recognition and targeting by antitumor CTLs (Seavey and Paterson, 2009).The epitope spreading phenomenon is further explained in Fig. 6.3. Thus, targeting endothelial cells through FLK-1 could induce epitope spreading to an endogenous tumor protein and lead to tumor death.

Targeting a molecule, such as FLK-1, which is expressed on normal vasculature arouses safety concerns of an autoimmune reaction that could damage normal vasculature. Although we saw no impact of the FLK-1 expressing *Listeria* vaccines on wound healing or gestation in mice, we sought a more precise angiogenic target for tumor vasculature. One promising molecule found specifically on tumor vasculature is endoglin (CD105), a member of the TGF-β receptor complex expressed on vascular endothelium and believed to play a role in angiogenesis. The importance of neovascularization during tumorigenesis is well characterized and CD105 is believed to be one of the factors involved in this process (Düwel *et al.*, 2007; Perez-Gomez *et al.*, 2007). As a prognostic, CD105 protein can be detected in the serum of tumor-bearing patients, and the levels of serum CD105 increase with metastatic severity (Li *et al.*, 2000; Takahashi *et al.*, 2001). Additionally, immunohistochemical analyses suggest that CD105 is highly expressed in the vascular endothelium of tumor tissue while it is barely detectable in the cognate normal tissues (Burrows

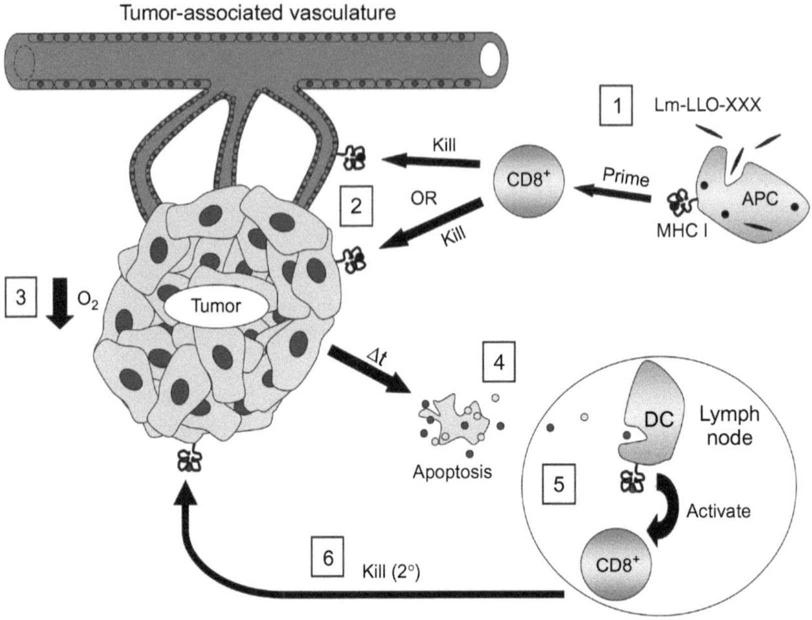

FIGURE 6.3 Targeting the tumor or tumor vasculature using *Listeria*-based vaccines can overcome tolerance and drive epitope spreading to cryptic tumor epitopes. (1) An Lm vaccine infects an antigen-presenting cell (APC) and primes autoreactive $CD8^+$ T cells to kill tumor or tumor-associated vascular cells expressing the cloned target ("XXX" may represent HPV16 E7, CD105, FLK-1, etc.); (2) elicited $CD8^+$ T cells attack and destroy the tumor or tumor vasculature; (3) destruction of key cells involved in maintaining the integrity of the tumor vasculature leads to increased tumor hypoxia and apoptosis; (4) apoptotic tumor cells are phagocytosed by resident dendritic cells (DC) in tumor-draining lymph nodes and cross-present tumor proteins to naive $CD8^+$ T cells; (5) due to the inflammatory milieu Lm induces, newly primed $CD8^+$ T cells targeting cryptic tumor epitopes are generated and migrate back to the inflamed tumor site; (6) resulting in a second wave of tumor cell killing. Note this model requires that both targets express the appropriate antigen-expressing molecules, MHC I. Downregulation of MHC I may increase NK cell activity, but immunosuppressive molecules and anti-NK proteins secreted by the tumor cells, like HLA-G, may prevent both mechanisms. (See Color Insert.)

et al., 1995; Wang *et al.*, 1993). Thus, targeting tumor-specific CD105 expression could possibly target tumor vasculature while sparing normal tissue. Preventive vaccination against CD105 has met with some success in controlling tumor growth (Lee *et al.*, 2006). We thus constructed two novel therapeutic vaccines, Lm-LLO-CD105A and Lm-LLO-CD105B, which included most of the molecule, directed against CD105 as a strategy to target neovascularization of established tumors and tested these for their therapeutic efficacy against primary and metastatic tumors in murine models for breast cancers. *Listeria*-based vaccines directed against these fragments of CD105 lead to therapeutic responses in mouse models of breast cancer, which was associated with a reduction of tumor vascularity. In the transgenic mouse model for autochthonous HER-2/neu-driven breast cancer, Lm-LLO-CD105A vaccination prevented the occurrence of breast tumors as well, if not better, than other vaccines we have constructed that target either the tumor antigen HER-2/neu or vascular endothelial cells. In comparison with previous *Listeria*-based vaccines targeting tumor vasculature, Lm-LLO-CD105A and Lm-LLO-CD105B demonstrated equivalent or superior efficacy against several mouse models of breast cancer.

Destroying only endothelial cells has limitations, however, since tumors can survive with limited numbers of endothelial cells. However, tumor vasculature is critically dependent on other cells, called mural pericytes. Pericytes act as support cells for capillaries and support the normal function and integrity of vasculature. Pericyte loss is associated with loss of vessel integrity, leading to eventual tissue starvation and hypoxia. Pericyte coverage of tumor vasculature is sparse; thus a further reduction in the numbers of these important cells could lead to the malfunctioning of mature blood vessels as the tumor grows in size.

As a blood vessel grows, pericytes arise from the vascular smooth muscle cells. Pericytes express a specialized glycoprotein, high-molecular weight melanoma-associated antigen (HMW-MAA) that interacts intimately with the extracellular matrix and is responsible for binding VEGF-A, MMPs, and bFGF. Originally identified on melanoma, human HMW-MAA is a cell surface, highly glycosylated, proteoglycan that is overexpressed on over 90% of benign nevi and melanoma lesions (Campoli *et al.*, 2004). Three different regions of the HMW-MAA molecule were cloned into *Listeria* fused to the truncated LLO molecule. Only one out of the three cloned molecules showed any efficacy; *Listeria*-LLO–HMW-MAA-C vaccine was able to slow the growth of transplanted B16F10 mouse melanoma cells in a subcutaneous model and eradicate primary breast tumors and lung metastases in a mouse model for breast cancer (Maciag *et al.*, 2008). In addition, the vaccine induced a significant reduction in tumor volume, MVD, and pericyte coverage, which correlated with an increase in $CD8^+$ cell infiltration into the tumor microenvironment. This vaccine failed to make a significant impact on pregnancy and wound healing in mice (Maciag *et al.*, 2008), indicating that it had few adverse effects.

5. *LISTERIA* AS A VECTOR FOR CDNA AND MRNA DELIVERY

L. monocytogenes has also been employed to deliver antigen-encoding cDNA by bactofection. Bactofection is a term used to describe the delivery of eukaryotic expression systems to mammalian cells utilizing bacteria as the vector (Dietrich *et al.*, 1998). Bactofection is a relatively new technology that takes advantage of the ability of facultative intracellular bacteria to be phagocytosed selectively by APCs. Once taken up by the cell, the bacterium is engineered to lyse and deliver its antigen-encoding cDNA to the cytosol. The delivered cDNA then translocates to the nucleus where it is transcribed and the antigen expressed and presented to the immune system by the APC. The advantage of using intracellular bacteria to deliver cDNA in antitumor immune therapy, therefore, comes from selective delivery of cDNA to APCs for efficient processing of tumor antigens and effective costimulatory molecule production in response to the *Listeria* infection. It could further eliminate the problems entailed by using a prokaryotic organism to deliver eukaryotic protein antigens. These include problems in expressing and secreting large and/or hydrophobic proteins and the lack of mechanisms for posttranslational modifications common in eukaryotic proteins and are discussed in more detail below.

Bactofection by *L. monocytogenes* was initially developed by Goebel and colleagues utilizing an attenuated *Listeria* strain that expressed a suicide cassette upon entering the cytosol of an infected host cell (Dietrich *et al.*, 1998; Spreng *et al.*, 2000). The suicide cassette consists of a phage lysin under the regulation of the cytosol-specific *actA* promoter. Once *Listeria* escapes the confines of the phagosome and enters the cytosol, expression of the phage lysin leads to the death of the bacterium and release of the cDNA plasmid to the cytosol. The cytosolic cDNA plasmid is then transferred to the nucleus instead of being degraded within the phagolysosome. Earlier bactofection vectors without a suicide cassette were still able to deliver cDNA that resulted in gene expression but with much lower efficiency. While initial optimization studies only involved the delivery of cDNA encoding for a reporter gene, eGFP, the *Listeria* bactofected cells were able to efficiently express and present the antigen, as measured by their ability to stimulate eGFP-specific $CD8^+$ T cells (Dietrich *et al.*, 1998; Spreng *et al.*, 2000).

While bactofection of plasmid DNA by *L. monocytogenes* demonstrated effectiveness for *in vitro* $CD8^+$ T cell stimulation, the results are less impressive in terms of *in vivo* effectiveness in a cervical cancer model (Souders *et al.*, 2006). In a direct comparison of *L. monocytogenes* strains that endogenously expressed and secreted the HPV-16 tumor antigen as protein (Gunn *et al.*, 2001) with DNA delivery strains, the latter proved a great deal less effective in stimulating antitumor immune responses *in vivo* (Souders *et al.*, 2006). The decreased effectiveness of *Listeria*-delivered plasmid DNA vaccines was hypothesized to be due to the relatively late expression of the tumor antigen, because of the need for transcription and translation (reviewed by Schoen *et al.*, 2008). In an effort to expedite the expression of the tumor antigen, a delivery system of translation-competent mRNA encoding for model tumor antigens by *Listeria* strains was developed (Loeffler *et al.*, 2006). Similar to the plasmid DNA delivery system, the mRNA strains contained a suicide cassette that would initiate the destruction of the *Listeria* vector upon entry of the bacterium into the cytosol. However, instead of releasing plasmid DNA upon lysis, the mRNA strains released T7 polymerase transcribed mRNA that contained an IRES element rendering it translation-competent in the eukaryotic host cell. This allowed for earlier expression of the tumor antigen to coincide with the infection, and ultimately, this augmented *in vivo* antitumor immune responses in direct comparison to a plasmid DNA delivery strain. However, while the mRNA delivery system was more effective than the plasmid DNA delivery strain, it was still not as effective as the *Listeria* strains that endogenously expressed and secreted the tumor antigen as a protein (Loeffler *et al.*, 2006). Clearly, further research is required before the potential of DNA/RNA delivery by *Listeria* reaches its full potential.

6. *LISTERIA* VIRULENCE FACTORS AS PROTEIN CARRIERS

6.1. LLO as an adjuvant

In addition to using *Listeria* as a vaccine vector, several other immunization strategies have arisen in our attempts to optimize the immunological impact of our vaccines while retaining a margin of safety. For example, the virulence factor LLO appears to have adjuvant-like properties. LLO is a 529 amino acid protein that is secreted by *L. monocytogenes* and mediates escape from the phagosome. We have found that fusion of a tumor antigen to the first 420 aa or so of LLO, which excludes the hemolytic domain, may facilitate secretion of the antigen (Gunn *et al.*, 2001; Ikonomidis *et al.*, 1994) increase antigen presentation (Sewell *et al.*, 2004b) and help to stimulate the maturation of DCs (Peng *et al.*, 2004). We have also shown that LLO can act as a potent adjuvant when incorporated into DNA vaccines (Peng *et al.*, 2007) or delivered by vaccinia virus rather than *Listeria* (Lamikanra *et al.*, 2001). These studies suggest that fusion of target tumor antigens directly to LLO in a recombinant protein-based vaccine may overcome the need for using whole live bacteria and perhaps lead to safer vaccine strategies.

We applied this approach to develop an immunotherapeutic for follicular lymphoma (FL), a low-grade B-cell lymphoma with an indolent clinical course where the disease increases in frequency with age. Treatment for FL has changed recently with the addition of Rituximab to the chemotherapy regimen (Marcus *et al.*, 2005). Consequently, patients with FL have an improved prognosis; however, they eventually relapse. A cancer vaccine approach to FL has long been the subject of study, with focus maintained on the possibility of inducing an immune response to the unique BCR idiotype of the transformed B cell that generated the lymphoma.

Idiotype-based vaccines, in which the BCR idiotype is conjugated to keyhole limpet hemocyanin (KLH) and delivered with GM-CSF, were originally tested in lymphoma mouse models but are now in phase III clinical trials for the treatment of FL. Idiotype-based vaccines have the potential to complement therapy-induced disease remission since the vaccine can act against minimal residual disease and induce memory to provide ongoing immunosurveillance. The use of KLH as the protein carrier for the BCR antigen dates back to the earliest studies investigating this approach in the 1980s (Kaminski *et al.*, 1986), and its choice was largely based on its even earlier use as a protein carrier to study humoral hapten responses. We, thus, investigated whether LLO could also assist an immune response against lymphoma idiotype protein and whether it was more effective than KLH. We found that Id-LLO better protected against challenge with a mouse lymphoma than Id-KLH. The tumor protection immunization protocol incorporating Id-LLO + mGM-CSF induced high-titer antiidiotype antibodies (with an increased ratio of IgG2a:IgG1 after one immunization) and this level persisted. *In vitro* studies showed a Th1 response and $CD4^+$ T cell proliferation in response to LLO or Id protein. In contrast, Id-KLH took two immunizations to reach the same titer of anti-Id antibodies, and the ratio of IgG2a:IgG1 was less than that obtained following Id-LLO immunization. The higher levels of IgG2a induced by Id-LLO may contribute to its greater efficacy since IgG2a anti-Id antibodies have been previously shown to induce higher levels of antibody-dependent cellular cytotoxicity activity against the mouse lymphoma than IgG1 anti-Id antibodies (Kaminski *et al.*, 1986). $CD4^+$ T cell proliferation in response to the Id antigen was equivalent between Id-LLO and Id-KLH; however, the proliferative response to KLH was less than that obtained for LLO. Since the function of the carrier protein is to provide $CD4^+$ T cell help for humoral responses to the Id antigen, these data suggest that LLO better served this purpose than KLH.

A major drawback in anti-Id tumor immunotherapy is the emergence of lymphoma cells that have lost BCR expression (Maloney *et al.*, 1992). This problem can be overcome if vaccine-mediated killing of the tumor cell induces epitope spreading to other tumor antigens (Cha *et al.*, 2006). To determine if mice vaccinated with our Id-based vaccines had mounted immune responses to antigens other than the Id antigen, surviving mice, from the two lymphoma challenge studies described above, were challenged with a BCR loss variant of the tumor. Mice immunized with Id-LLO showed better rejection of this variant than those immunized with Id-KLH. However, this improved survival was only present after the mice had been challenged twice with the parent lymphoma, that is, epitope spreading in this setting required two challenges with the parental lymphoma cells.

These studies showed that the vaccine conjugate Id-LLO induced a powerful humoral and $CD4^+$ T cell-mediated response dominated by a

Th1 phenotype and compares favorably to Id-KLH in tumor protection studies against an aggressive mouse lymphoma (Campbell *et al.*, 1990; Kwak *et al.*, 1990) The utility of LLO as an adjuvant for protein-based vaccines has been confirmed in other, unpublished, studies where we investigated the use of LLO as an adjuvant for the HPV-16 E7 protein in our cervical cancer models described above. We found that recombinant E7 protein either mixed with LLO or as a genetic fusion was effective at eradicating the TC-1 tumor implanted into mice. The molecular basis of LLO's adjuvant properties is at present unclear. Originally, we thought it was due to the presence of a PEST sequence at its amino terminus, which augments proteosomal degradation (Decatur and Portnoy, 2000). However, this work was later called into question (Schnupf *et al.*, 2006). Nevertheless, removal or addition of the PEST sequence from LLO fused to the tumor antigen correlates with changes in effective tumor immunotherapy and $CD8^+$ T cell induction (Sewell *et al.*, 2004b). Previous studies by other laboratories have attributed its potency to its hemolytic properties (Bahey-El-Din *et al.*, 2010; Nitcheu-Tefit, *et al.*, 2007; Radford *et al.*, 2002), but in our work, because of the cellular toxicity of LLO, we have abrogated this property by either truncating the molecule and removing the hemolytic domain or by mutating the cholesterol-binding site. Rather, we believe it is acting as a classical PAMP. PAMPs are recognized by specific pathogen-recognition receptors that activate an immunostimulatory cascade leading to the release of proinflammatory cytokines such as TNF-alpha and IL-12 (D'Andrea *et al.*, 1992; Hartmann and Krieg, 1999; Klinman *et al.*, 1996). These critically important cytokines facilitate the maturation of APCs and the activation of antigen-specific CTLs (Biron and Gazzinelli, 1995; Wolf *et al.*, 1994). We have evidence that LLO may be involved in the maturation of DCs (Peng *et al.*, 2004), which supports our hypothesis that LLO acts as a PAMP.

6.2. ActA as an adjuvant

On examining the sequence of the *Listeria*-derived virulence factor, ActA, we discovered several PEST sequences and thus decided to test its ability to act as an adjuvant for tumor immunotherapy. We constructed a *Listeria* recombinant similar to our Lm-LLO antigen constructs but replacing the coding region of LLO with the first 390 residues of ActA, which includes all four of the PEST sequences found in the molecule (Sewell *et al.*, 2004a, 2008). As we described above, Lm-ActA-E7 was as effective as Lm-LLO-E7 as a tumor immunotherapeutic in eradicating transplanted HPV-transformed tumors in the wild-type mouse (Sewell *et al.*, 2004a) in the mouse transgenic for HPV-16 E7 described above (Souders *et al.*, 2007) and also in impacting on the growth of autochthonous tumors in the E7 transgenic mouse (Sewell *et al.*, 2008).

We, thus, investigated the ability of ActA protein to act as an adjuvant in a protein-based vaccine strategy with recombinant E7 protein. For this, we used a gene encoding for amino acids 25–421 of the ActA protein and expressed it from *E. coli* either as a fusion protein with E7 (ActA-E7) or alone (Wood *et al.*, 2010). We then tested ActA-E7 and a mixture of ActA and E7 for their antitumor properties compared to E7 alone and found that ActA either fused to or administered as a mixture with a tumor antigen can augment antitumor immune responses, break immune tolerance in the E7 transgenic mouse, and facilitate tumor eradication in a $CD8^+$ T cell-dependent manner. This suggests that ActA is not only an effective adjuvant in tumor immunotherapy but can also be applied in a number of therapeutic settings. This study also demonstrated that, similar to LLO, ActA does not need to be secreted by *Listeria* or fused to the tumor-specific antigen in order to gain the benefits of its adjuvant properties. We thus believe that, like LLO, ActA could be facilitating antitumor immune responses by acting as a PAMP, similar to other bacterial adjuvants such as CPG and LPS (D'Andrea *et al.*, 1992; Hartmann and Krieg, 1999; Klinman *et al.*, 1996). PAMPs are used widely in tumor immunotherapy to facilitate strong cell mediated antitumor immune responses similar to those induced by ActA vaccination. We are currently investigating whether ActA has PAMP properties.

7. DIRECT TUMOR KILLING BY *LISTERIA*

In collaboration with our laboratory, Dr. Claudia Gravekamp recently made the interesting finding that *Listeria* can infect and kill mouse and human breast tumor cells *in vitro* and primary breast tumors and metastases *in vivo* (Kim *et al.*, 2009). At this point, it is not clear which receptors on the tumor cells facilitate invasion by *Listeria*. However, an intriguing candidate is E-cadherin, the receptor to which the *Listeria* surface virulence factor inlA binds and which is highly expressed in many cancers including breast cancer (Kowalski *et al.*, 2003).

The presence of bacteria in tumor cells has been previously observed (Stritzker *et al.*, 2008; Velge *et al.*, 1994; Yu *et al.*, 2004). Yu *et al.* (2004) have shown that attenuated pathogens, such as *Vibrio cholera*, and *S. typhimurium*, enter tumors and metastases followed by replication. In this same study, they demonstrated that an attenuated *Listeria* carrying a green fluorescence protein infects human prostate tumor cells in a xenograft model *in vivo*. In addition, Stritzker *et al.* (2008) have shown that an attenuated *Listeria* infects tumor cells. However, in contrast to the discovery of the Gravekamp lab, neither did they report *Listeria*-induced killing of the infected tumors nor did they investigate the mechanism by which bacteria can cause the death of tumor cells.

It is known that bacteria can trigger apoptosis through a large variety of mechanisms that include the secretion of protein synthesis inhibitors, pore forming proteins, or molecules responsible for the activation of the endogenous death machinery in infected cells (Lancellotti *et al.*, 2006). However, the novel mechanism by which *Listeria* kills tumor cells is through the activation of nicotinamide adenine dinucleotide phosphate (NADPH) oxidase and the subsequent production of ROS (Kim *et al.*, 2009). The Gravekamp lab demonstrated the involvement of NADPH oxidase-mediated ROS in tumor cell death, using Trolox, a scavenger of OH• radicals, and apocynin or diphenylene iodonium (DPI). Both selective inhibitors of NADPH oxidase prevented 50% of the *Listeria*-induced tumor cell death. They also demonstrated with live cell microscopy and H_2DFFDA or CM-H_2XRos that cytosolic ROS were produced through activated NADPH oxidase and that mitochondrial ROS were produced as well. LLO is known to be involved in the rapid increase in intracellular Ca^{2+} levels upon infection of the macrophage cell line, J774, by *Listeria* (Wadsworth and Goldfine, 2002). Kim *et al.* (2009) found that *Listeria* increased intracellular Ca^{2+} levels resulting in the production of high levels of mROS. These results imply that NADPH oxidase and excessive intracellular calcium contribute to tumor cell death upon LM-LLO infection causing mitochondrial failure.

The ability of *Listeria* to directly kill tumor cells clearly adds to the mechanisms by which *Listeria* controls tumor growth. The findings of the Gravekamp lab also open up the possibility of using *Listeria* as a tumor-homing vector for prodrugs or other cancer therapeutics.

8. CHALLENGES IN MOVING *LISTERIA*-BASED TUMOR IMMUNOTHERAPY INTO THE CLINIC

The use of vaccine strains of *Listeria* for cancer immunotherapy has moved from the research laboratory to clinical trials with treatment for cervical, breast, and prostate cancer in humans under development. After almost 10 years of preclinical development, Lm-LLO-E7, the *Listeria* vaccine that secretes an LLO-E7 fusion product (Gunn *et al.*, 2001) entered clinical trials. The results of the clinical phase I safety study of Lm-LLO-E7 showed that vaccinations were safe for use in patients with late-stage invasive carcinoma of the cervix (Maciag *et al.*, 2009). All of the 15 patients enrolled experienced flu-like symptoms which were alleviated by non-prescription symptomatic treatment. Although the study was not designed to evaluate efficacy, more than half of the patients treated with the vaccine had stable disease and one patient was considered a partial responder. The median survival was 347 days for all the patients and almost 4 years for two patients. Table 6.3 shows the survival data for

TABLE 6.3 Most recent median and mean survival of patients treated with Lm-LLO-E7 in the study earlier reported and described in Maciag *et al.* (2009) (updated data courtesy of Dr. Jon Rothman, Advaxis Inc.)

Dosage group	Patient #	Study day 1	Date of death	Study day at death	Days alive as of 1/1/2011
1×10^9	01-001	4-Apr-06	6-Apr-07	367	
	01-002	26-Apr-06	22-Aug-06	118	
	01-003	10-May-06	22-Apr-07	347	
	01-004	5-Oct-06			1549
	04-001	28-Aug-06	13-Sep-07	381	
3.3×10^9	03-001	14-Dec-06	2-Nov-07	323	
	04-002	26-Oct-06	13-Apr-08	535	
	04-003	6-Nov-06	5-Oct-09	1064	
	04-004	14-Dec-06	11-Mar-07	87	
	04-005	14-Dec-06	19-Jan-07	36	
1×10^{10}	01-005	14-Feb-07	11-Aug-07	178	
	01-006	31-Jan-07	13-Aug-07	194	
	01-007	13-Feb-07			1418
	02-006	15-Mar-07	11-Dec-07	Lost to	follow-up
	04-006	15-Feb-07	10-Aug-08	542	
	Median survival			347	
	Mean survival			485	

N.B. Patient 02-2006 was lost to follow-up. Her last contact date was on day 271. The study was closed on 01/01/2011.

patients that entered this study as of the end of 2010 when follow-up was terminated. Fifty-three percent of patients survived more than 1 year compared to 5% of patients who receive conventional treatment. These are remarkable results compared to historical controls since the median survival time of patients with previously treated metastatic, refractory, or recurrent cervical cancer is only 6–7 months (Moore *et al.*, 2010). This study showed for the first time that a live-attenuated *Listeria* immunotherapeutic is safe to be administered to late-stage invasive cancer patients and may provide some efficacy. This immunotherapeutic is now in four phase 2 clinical trials; two are for advanced cervical cancer in the United States and in India, one is for cervical intraepithelial neoplasia (an early noninvasive form of cervical cancer) that will take place in the United States, and the fourth is for HPV-associated head and neck cancer in the UK (http://www.advaxis.com/page/pipeline.html). At the time of writing, over 100 patients have been dosed with this *Listeria* vector with no serious adverse events. In addition, Advaxis Inc. anticipates starting a phase I trial using Lm-LLO-PSA*ddA* (Wallecha *et al.*, 2009b) for prostate cancer and Lm-LLO-chHER-2/*neuddA* (Shahabi *et al.*, 2011) for breast cancer next year.

Despite the great advances made in the development of *Listeria*-based vaccines for cancer treatment, there are still a number of safety, technical, and biological challenges. The *Listeria* vector, Lm-LLO-E7, although showing great promise in clinical trials is not the ideal host strain for use in humans. It carries a chloramphenicol antibiotic resistance gene on its plasmid required to select the transformed bacterium *in vitro*. The FDA discourages the presence of any antibiotic resistance genes in vaccines because of concerns of the possibility of environmental spread of the vector. This selection mechanism has been replaced in later constructs by an alanine racemase selection mechanism that removes the necessity for antibiotic resistance (Verch *et al.*, 2004). The use of live pathogen-based vectors always raises concerns about safety in potentially immunocompromised cancer patients. To avoid adverse events, suitably attenuated strains should be used and patients should be screened for immune deficiencies prior to treatment. However, bacteria have an advantage over viral vectors because of the availability of a wide range of antibiotics that can be used to curtail infection. Thus, potential adverse events can be avoided by the application of a suitable antibiotic before the bacterial infection is beyond control. Most of the safety concerns raised for *Listeria*-based vectors, such as the possibility of bacterial meningitis, can easily be addressed this way. In addition, an antibiotic regimen should be included in clinical protocols with live bacterial vectors at the assumed end of the vector infection for safety reasons.

Concerns are also often raised about the possibility of *Listeria* contagion from the patient to healthcare workers or the patient's family although person-to-person transmission of *Listeria* has not been documented even in clinically confirmed cases of listeriosis (Bennet Lorber, personal communication). The rational attenuation of virulence factors can reduce concerns about pathogenicity while still maintaining a vector with the required immune properties. To further reduce the pathogenicity of the most recently developed constructs, the ActA gene was deleted. These improved vectors appear to be as effective in cancer immunotherapy (Shahabi *et al.*, 2011; Wallecha *et al.*, 2009b).

There are many technical challenges surrounding the expression and secretion of eukaryotic proteins by bacteria. Bacteria are unable to carry out a variety of posttranslational protein modifications observed in mammalian cells limiting the pool of TAAs that can serve as the basis of bacterial vaccine constructs. Very hydrophobic regions of the passenger antigen can be poorly secreted, and there is a size limit of about 60 kDa greater than which we observe reduced expression and secretion. We have overcome this by selecting regions of the molecule more likely to contain human CTL epitopes (HMW-MAA, VEGF, CD105) or by creating several vectors each of which expresses overlapping fragments of the whole antigen (HER-2/neu). In addition, the expression of foreign antigens in bacteria can place a metabolic burden on the organism that can affect growth rate and select for plasmid loss in the case of plasmid-transformed bacteria or mutant bacteria that have shut down antigen expression (Galan and Levine, 2001; Peters and Paterson, 2003). The issue of plasmid loss can be addressed by a complementation system where a gene required by the bacterium for survival *in vivo* is deleted from its chromosome and included on the plasmid to complement for this loss (Ikonomidis *et al.*, 1994; Verch *et al.*, 2004). Nevertheless, there are some TAAs, which we have simply found it impossible to express by *Listeria* even *in vitro*. Fortunately, there are a number of candidate antigens for every cancer from which to select a target that is suitable for expression and secretion by *Listeria*.

Another concern in using a ubiquitous pathogen found in nature, such as *Listeria* as a vaccine vector, is the degree of exposure the population has had to the wild-type pathogen, which could compromise the infection rate of vaccine strains. Since it is a relatively mild pathogen, there has never been a vaccination program directed against *Listeria*, *per se*, as there has against other potential vectors such as vaccinia virus and *Salmonella*. Nevertheless, there has been public exposure by natural infection such that 60% of normal healthy adults have circulating LLO-specific T cells (Leong *et al.*, 2009). Nevertheless, although mice with preexisting cellular immunity to *L. monocytogenes* displayed attenuated $CD8^+$ T cell responses to recombinant strains of *Listeria* expressing a target antigen such as OVA, this could be overcome by repeated immunizations (Leong *et al.*, 2009). In addition, *Listeria* expressing a TAA has been shown to be an effective tumor immunotherapeutic in mice previously immunized with wild-type *L. monocytogenes* (Starks *et al.*, 2004). Thus, at least in hosts with intact immune system, some preexisting immunity may not limit the use of *Listeria* as a therapeutic in clinical settings.

Despite these many challenges to designing and constructing the "perfect" *L. monocytogenes* cancer vaccine vector, given the promise that *Listeria* has displayed as a cancer immunotherapeutic in preclinical and clinical studies, it is worth pursuing solutions to these obstacles.

ACKNOWLEDGMENT

Yvonne Paterson wishes to disclose that she has a financial interest in Advaxis, Inc., a vaccine and therapeutic company that has licensed or has an option to license all patents from the University of Pennsylvania that concern the use of *Listeria* or listerial products as vaccines.

REFERENCES

Anderson, M. S., Venanzi, E. S., Klein, L., Chen, Z., Berzins, S. P., Turley, S. J., von Boehmer, H., Bronson, R., Dierich, A., Benoist, C., and Mathis, D. (2002). Projection of an immunological self shadow within the thymus by the aire protein. *Science* **298,** 1395–1401.

Anderson, M. S., Venanzi, E. S., Chen, Z., Berzins, S. P., Benoist, C., and Mathis, D. (2005). The cellular mechanism of Aire control of T cell tolerance. *Immunity* **23,** 227–239.

Bahey-El-Din, M., Casey, P. G., Griffin, B. T., and Gahan, C. G. (2010). Expression of two Listeria monocytogenes antigens (P60 and LLO) in Lactococcus lactis and examination for use as live vaccine vectors. *J. Med. Microbiol.* **59,** 904–912.

Beatty, G. L., and Paterson, Y. (2001). Regulation of tumor growth by IFN-gamma in cancer immunotherapy. *Immunol. Res.* **24,** 201–210.

Biron, C. A., and Gazzinelli, R. T. (1995). Effects of IL-12 on immune responses to microbial infections, a key mediator in regulating disease outcome. *Curr. Opin. Immunol.* **7,** 485–496.

Brockstedt, D. G., Giedlin, M. A., Leong, M. L., Bahjat, K. S., Gao, Y., Luckett, W., Liu, W., Cook, D. N., Portnoy, D. A., and Dubensky, T. W., Jr. (2004). *Listeria*-based cancer vaccines that segregate immunogenicity from toxicity. *Proc. Natl. Acad. Sci. USA* **101,** 13832–13837.

Bruhn, K. W., Craft, N., Nguyen, B. D., Yip, J., and Miller, J. F. (2005). Characterization of anti-self CD8 T-cell responses stimulated by recombinant *Listeria monocytogenes* expressing the melanoma antigen TRP-2. *Vaccine* **23,** 4263–4272.

Brzoza, K. L., Rockel, A. B., and Hiltbold, E. M. (2004). Cytoplasmic entry of Listeria monocytogenes enhances dendritic cell maturation and T cell differentiation and function. *J. Immunol.* **173,** 2641–2651.

Burrows, F. J., Derbyshire, E. J., Tazzari, P. L., Amlot, P., Gazdar, A. F., King, S. W., Letarte, M., Vitetta, E. S., and Thorpe, P. E. (1995). Up-regulation of endoglin on vascular endothelial cells in human solid tumors, implications for diagnosis and therapy. *Clin. Cancer Res.* **1,** 1623–1634.

Campbell, M. J., Esserman, L., Byars, N. E., Allison, A. C., and Levy, R. (1990). Idiotype vaccination against murine B cell lymphoma. Humoral and cellular requirements for the full expression of antitumor immunity. *J. Immunol.* **145,** 1029–1036.

Campoli, M. R., Chang, C. C., Kageshita, T., Wang, X., McCarthy, J. B., and Ferrone, S. (2004). Human high molecular weight-melanoma-associated antigen (HMW-MAA), a melanoma cell surface chondroitin sulfate proteoglycan (MSCP) with biological and clinical significance. *Crit. Rev. Immunol.* **24,** 267–296.

Cha, S. C., Kwak, L. W., Ruffini, P. A., Qin, H., Neelapu, S., and Biragyn, A. (2006). Cloning of B cell lymphoma-associated antigens using modified phage-displayed expression cDNA library and immunized patient sera. *J. Immunol. Methods* **312,** 79–93.

Chang, H. L., Gillett, N., Figari, I., Lopez, A. R., Palladino, M. A., and Derynck, R. (1993). Increased transforming growth factor beta expression inhibits cell proliferation in vitro, yet increases tumorigenicity and tumor growth of Meth A sarcoma cells. *Cancer Res.* **53,** 4391–4398.

Coley, W. B. (1893). The treatment of malignant tumors by repeated inoculations of erysipelas, with a report of ten original cases. *Am. J. Med. Sci.* **105,** 487–511.

Coley, W. B. (1909). The treatment of inoperable sarcoma by bacterial toxins (the mixed toxins of the streptococcus of erysipelas and the bacillus prodigiosus). *Practitioner* **83,** 589–613.

D'Andrea, A., Rengaraju, M., Valiante, N. M., Chehimi, J., Kubin, M., Aste, M., Chan, S. H., Kobayashi, M., Young, D., and Nickbarg, E. (1992). Production of natural killer cell stimulatory factor (interleukin 12) by peripheral blood mononuclear cells. *J. Exp. Med.* **176,** 1387–1398.

Decatur, A. L., and Portnoy, D. A. (2000). A PEST-like sequence in listeriolysin O essential for Listeria monocytogenes pathogenicity. *Science* **290,** 992–995.

Derbinski, J., Schulte, A., Kyewski, B., and Klein, L. (2001). Promiscuous gene expression in medullary thymic epithelial cells mirrors the peripheral self. *Nat. Immunol.* **2,** 1032–1039.

Dietrich, G., Bubert, A., Gentschev, I., Sokolovic, Z., Simm, A., Catic, A., Kaufmann, S. H., Hess, J., Szalay, A. A., and Goebel, W. (1998). Delivery of antigen-encoding plasmid DNA into the cytosol of macrophages by attenuated suicide *Listeria monocytogenes. Nat. Biotechnol.* **16,** 181–185.

Dominiecki, M. E., Beatty, G. L., Pan, Z. K., Neeson, P., and Paterson, Y. (2005). Tumor sensitivity to IFN-gamma is required for successful antigen-specific immunotherapy of a transplantable mouse tumor model for HPV-transformed tumors. *Cancer Immunol. Immunother.* **54,** 477–488.

Drake, C. G., Jaffee, E., and Pardoll, D. M. (2006). Mechanisms of immune evasion by tumors. *Adv. Immunol.* **90,** 51–81.

Düwel, A., Eleno, N., Jerkic, M., Arevalo, M., Bolaños, J. P., Bernabeu, C., and López-Novoa, J. M. (2007). Reduced tumor growth and angiogenesis in endoglin-haploinsufficient mice. *Tumour Biol.* **28,** 1–8.

Ercolini, A. M., Machiels, J. P., Chen, Y. C., Slansky, J. E., Giedlen, M., Reilly, R. T., and Jaffee, E. M. (2003). Identification and characterization of the immunodominant rat HER-2/neu MHC class I epitope presented by spontaneous mammary tumors from HER-2/neu-transgenic mice. *J. Immunol.* **170,** 4273–4280.

Folkman, J. (1971). Tumor angiogenesis, therapeutic implications. *N. Engl. J. Med.* **285,** 1182–1186.

Folkman, J. (1996). Tumor angiogenesis and tissue factor. *Nat. Med.* **2,** 167–168.

Galan, J. E., and Levine, M. M. (2001). Can a "flawless" live vector vaccine strain be engineered? *Trends Microbiol.* **9,** 372–376.

Gallegos, A. M., and Bevan, M. J. (2004). Central tolerance to tissue-specific antigens mediated by direct and indirect antigen presentation. *J. Exp. Med.* **200,** 1039–1049.

Gillison, M. L., Koch, W. M., Capone, R. B., Spafford, M., Westra, W. H., Wu, L., Zahurak, M. L., Daniel, R. W., Viglione, M., Symer, D. E., Shah, K. V., and Sidransky, D. (2000). Evidence for a causal association between human papilloma virus and a subset of head and neck cancers. *J. Natl. Cancer Inst.* **92,** 709–720.

Gunn, G. R., Zubair, A., Peters, C., Pan, Z. K., Wu, T. C., and Paterson, Y. (2001). Two *Listeria monocytogenes* vaccine vectors that express different molecular forms of human papilloma virus-16 (HPV-16) E7 induce qualitatively different T cell immunity that correlates with their ability to induce regression of established tumors immortalized by HPV-16. *J. Immunol.* **167,** 6471–6479.

Hartmann, G., and Krieg, A. M. (1999). CpG DNA and LPS induce distinct patterns of activation in human monocytes. *Gene Ther.* **6,** 893–903.

Hu, J. K., Kagari, T., Clingan, J. M., and Matloubian, M. (2011). Expression of chemokine receptor CXCR3 on T cells affects the balance between effector and memory CD8 T-cell generation. *Proc. Natl. Acad. Sci. USA* **108,** E118–E127.

Huang, B., Zhao, J., Shen, S., Li, H., He, K. L., Shen, G. X., Mayer, L., Unkeless, J., Li, D., Yuan, Y., Zhang, G. M., Xiong, H., *et al.* (2007). *Listeria monocytogenes* promotes tumor growth via tumor cell toll-like receptor 2 signaling. *Cancer Res.* **67,** 4346–4352.

Hussain, S. F., and Paterson, Y. (2004). CD4+CD25+ regulatory T cells that secrete TGF-beta and IL-10 are preferentially induced by a vaccine vector. *J. Immunother.* **27,** 339–346.

Hussain, S. F., and Paterson, Y. (2005). What is needed for effective antitumor immunotherapy? Lessons learned using Listeria monocytogenes as a live vector for HPV-associated tumors. *Cancer Immunol. Immunother.* **54,** 577–586.

Ikonomidis, G., Paterson, Y., Kos, F. J., and Portnoy, D. A. (1994). Delivery of a viral antigen to the class I processing and presentation pathway by Listeria monocytogenes. *J. Exp. Med.* **180,** 2209–2218.

Ishizaki, H., Song, G. Y., Srivastava, T., Carroll, K. D., Shahabi, V., Manuel, E. R., Diamond, D. J., and Ellenhorn, J. D. (2010). Heterologous prime/boost immunization with p53-based vaccines combined with toll-like receptor stimulation enhances tumor regression. *J. Immunother.* **33,** 609–617.

Jensen, E. R., Selvakumar, R., Shen, H., Ahmed, R., Wettstein, F. O., and Miller, J. F. (1997). Recombinant *Listeria monocytogenes* vaccination eliminates papillomavirus-induced tumors and prevents papilloma formation from viral DNA. *J. Virol.* **71,** 8467–8474.

Kaminski, M. S., Kitamura, K., Maloney, D. G., Campbell, M. J., and Levy, R. (1986). Importance of antibody isotype in monoclonal anti-idiotype therapy of a murine B cell lymphoma. A study of hybridoma class switch variants. *J. Immunol.* **136,** 1123–1130.

Kim, S. H., Castro, F., Gonzalez, D., Maciag, P. C., Paterson, Y., and Gravekamp, C. (2008). Mage-b vaccine delivered by recombinant *Listeria monocytogenes* is highly effective against breast cancer metastases. *Br. J. Cancer* **99,** 741–749.

Kim, S. H., Castro, F., Paterson, Y., and Gravekamp, C. (2009). High efficacy of a *Listeria*-based vaccine against metastatic breast cancer reveals a dual mode of action. *Cancer Res.* **69,** 5860–5866.

Klinman, D. M., Yi, A. K., Beaucage, S. L., Conover, J., and Krieg, A. M. (1996). CpG motifs present in bacteria DNA rapidly induce lymphocytes to secrete interleukin 6, interleukin 12, and interferon gamma. *Proc. Natl. Acad. Sci. USA* **93,** 2879–2883.

Kolb-Mäurer, A., Gentschev, I., Fries, H. W., Fiedler, F., Bröcker, E. B., Kämpgen, E., and Goebel, W. (2000). Listeria monocytogenes-infected human dendritic cells, uptake and host cell response. *Infect. Immun.* **68,** 3680–3688.

Kowalski, P. J., Rubin, M. A., and Kleer, R. (2003). E-cadherin expression in primary carcinomas of the breast and its distant metastases. *Cancer Res.* **5,** R217–R222.

Kwak, L. W., Campbell, M. J., Zelenetz, A. D., and Levy, R. (1990). Combined syngeneic bone marrow transplantation and immunotherapy of a murine B-cell lymphoma, active immunization with tumor-derived idiotypic immunoglobulin. *Blood* **76,** 2411–2417.

Lamikanra, A., Pan, Z. K., Isaacs, S., Wu, T. C., and Paterson, Y. (2001). Regression of established Human Papillomavirus (HPV-16) immortalized tumors in vivo by vaccinia viruses expressing different forms of HPV-16 E7 correlates with enhanced $CD8^+$ T cell responses that home to the tumor site. *J. Virol.* **75,** 9654–9664.

Lancellotti, M., Brocchi, M., and da Silveira, W. D. (2006). Bacteria-induced apoptosis, an approach to bacterial pathogenesis. *Braz. J. Morphol. Sci.* **23,** 75–86.

Lee, S. H., Mizutani, N., Mizutani, M., Luo, Y., Zhou, H., Kaplan, C., Kim, S. W., Xiang, R., and Reisfeld, R. A. (2006). Endoglin (CD105) is a target for an oral DNA vaccine against breast cancer. *Cancer Immunol. Immunother.* **55,** 1565–1574.

Leong, M. L., Hampl, J., Liu, W., Mathur, S., Bahjat, K. S., Luckett, W., Dubensky, T. W., Jr., and Brockstedt, D. G. (2009). Impact of preexisting vector-specific immunity on vaccine potency, characterization of *Listeria monocytogenes*-specific humoral and cellular immunity in humans and modeling studies using recombinant vaccines in mice. *Infect. Immun.* **77,** 3958–3968.

Li, C., Guo, B., Wilson, P. B., Stewart, A., Byrne, G., Bundred, N., and Kumar, S. (2000). Plasma levels of soluble CD105 correlate with metastasis in patients with breast cancer. *Int. J. Cancer* **89,** 122–126.

Liau, L. M., Jensen, E. R., Kremen, T. J., Odesa, S. K., Sykes, S. N., Soung, M. C., Miller, J. F., and Bronstein, J. M. (2002). Tumor immunity within the central nervous system stimulated by recombinant *Listeria monocytogenes* vaccination. *Cancer Res.* **62,** 2287–2293.

Lin, K. Y., Guarnieri, F. G., Staveley-O'Carroll, K. F., Levitsky, H. I., August, T. J., Pardoll, D. M., and Wu, T. C. (1996). Treatment of established tumors with a novel vaccine that enhances major histocompatibility class II presentation of tumor antigen. *Cancer Res.* **56,** 21–26.

Lin, C. W., Lee, J. Y., Tsao, Y. P., Shen, C. P., Lai, H. C., and Chen, S. L. (2002). Oral vaccination with recombinant *Listeria monocytogenes* expressing human papillomavirus type 16 E7 can cause tumor growth in mice to regress. *Int. J. Cancer* **102,** 629–637.

Liston, A., Lesage, S., Wilson, J., Peltonen, L., and Goodnow, C. C. (2003). Aire regulates negative selection of organ-specific T cells. *Nat. Immunol.* **4,** 350–354.

Liston, A., Gray, D. H., Lesage, S., Fletcher, A. L., Wilson, J., Webster, K. E., Scott, H. S., Boyd, R. L., Peltonen, L., and Goodnow, C. C. (2004). Gene dosage-limiting role of Aire in thymic expression, clonal deletion, and organ-specific autoimmunity. *J. Exp. Med.* **200,** 1015–1026.

Loeffler, D. I., Schoen, C. U., Goebel, W., and Pilgrim, S. (2006). Comparison of different live vaccine strategies in vivo for delivery of protein antigen or antigen-encoding DNA and mRNA by virulence-attenuated *Listeria monocytogenes. Infect. Immun.* **74,** 3946–3957.

Lowy, D. R., Kirnbauer, R., and Schiller, J. T. (1994). Genital human papillomavirus infection. *Proc. Natl. Acad. Sci. USA* **91,** 2436–2440.

Luo, Y., Markowitz, D., Xiang, R., Zhou, H., and Reisfeld, R. A. (2007). FLK-1-based minigene vaccines induce T cell-mediated suppression of angiogenesis and tumor protective immunity in syngeneic BALB/c mice. *Vaccine* **25,** 1409–1415.

Maciag, P. C., Seavey, M. M., Pan, Z. K., Ferrone, S., and Paterson, Y. (2008). Cancer immunotherapy targeting the high molecular weight melanoma-associated antigen protein results in a broad antitumor response and reduction of pericytes in the tumor vasculature. *Cancer Res.* **68,** 8066–8075.

Maciag, P. C., Radulovic, S., and Rothman, J. (2009). The first clinical use of a live-attenuated *Listeria monocytogenes* vaccine, a phase I safety study of Lm-LLO-E7 in patients with advanced carcinoma of the cervix. *Vaccine* **27,** 3975–3983.

Maloney, D. G., Brown, S., Czerwinski, D. K., Liles, T. M., Hart, S. M., Miller, R. A., and Levy, R. (1992). Monoclonal anti-idiotype antibody therapy of B-cell lymphoma, the addition of a short course of chemotherapy does not interfere with the antitumor effect nor prevent the emergence of idiotype-negative variant cells. *Blood* **80,** 1502–1510.

Marcus, R., Imrie, K., Belch, A., Cunningham, D., Flores, E., Catalano, J., Solal-Celigny, P., Offner, F., Walewski, J., Raposo, J., Jack, A., and Smith, P. (2005). CVP chemotherapy plus rituximab compared with CVP as first-line treatment for advanced follicular lymphoma. *Blood* **105,** 1417–1423.

McCarthy, E. F. (2006). The toxins of William B. Coley and the treatment of bone and soft-tissue sarcomas. *Iowa Orthop. J.* **26,** 154–158.

Moore, D. H., Tian, C., Monk, B. J., Long, H. J., Omura, G. A., and Bloss, J. D. (2010). Prognostic factors for response to cisplatin-based chemotherapy in advanced cervical carcinoma, a Gynecologic Oncology Group Study. *Gynecol. Oncol.* **116,** 44–49.

Mustafa, W., Maciag, P. C., Pan, Z. K., Weaver, J. R., Xiao, Y., Isaacs, S. N., and Paterson, Y. (2009). *Listeria monocytogenes* delivery of HPV-16 major capsid protein L1 induces systemic and mucosal cell-mediated CD4+ and CD8+ T-cell responses after oral immunization. *Viral Immunol.* **22,** 195–204.

Niethammer, A. G., Xiang, R., Becker, J. C., Wodrich, H., Pertl, U., Karsten, G., Eliceiri, B. P., and Reisfeld, R. A. (2002). A DNA vaccine against VEGF receptor 2 prevents effective angiogenesis and inhibits tumor growth. *Nat. Med.* **8,** 1369–1375.

Nitcheu-Tefit, J., Dai, M. S., Critchley-Thorne, R. J., Ramirez-Jimenez, F., Xu, M., Conchon, S., Ferry, N., Stauss, H. J., and Vassaux, G. (2007). Listeriolysin O expressed in a bacterial vaccine suppresses CD4+CD25high regulatory T cell function in vivo. *J. Immunol.* **179,** 1532–1541.

Onizuka, S., Tawara, I., Shimizu, J., Sakaguchi, S., Fujita, T., and Nakayama, E. (1999). Tumor rejection by in vivo administration of anti-CD25 (interleukin-2 receptor alpha) monoclonal antibody. *Cancer Res.* **59,** 3128–3133.

Paglia, P., Arioli, I., Frahm, N., Chakraborty, T., Colombo, M. P., and Guzmàn, C. A. (1997). The defined attenuated Listeria monocytogenes delta mp12 mutant is an effective oral vaccine carrier to trigger a long-lasting immune response against a mouse fibrosarcoma. *Eur. J. Immunol.* **27,** 1570–1575.

Pamer, E. G., Sijts, A. J., Villanueva, M. S., Busch, D. H., and Vijh, S. (1997). MHC class I antigen processing of *Listeria monocytogenes* proteins, implications for dominant and subdominant CTL responses. *Immunol. Rev.* **158,** 129–136.

Pan, Z. K., Ikonomidis, G., Lazenby, A., Pardoll, D., and Paterson, Y. (1995a). A recombinant *Listeria monocytogenes* vaccine expressing a model tumour antigen protects mice against lethal tumour cell challenge and causes regression of established tumours. *Nat. Med.* **1,** 471–477.

Pan, Z. K., Ikonomidis, G., Pardoll, D., and Paterson, Y. (1995b). Regression of established tumors in mice mediated by the oral administration of a recombinant Listeria monocytogenes vaccine. *Cancer Res.* **55,** 4776–4779.

Pan, Z. K., Weiskirch, L. M., and Paterson, Y. (1999). Regression of established B16F10 melanoma with a recombinant *Listeria monocytogenes vaccine*. *Cancer Res.* **59,** 5264–5269.

Paterson, Y., Guirnalda, P. D., and Wood, L. M. (2010). Listeria and Salmonella bacterial vectors of tumor-associated antigens for cancer immunotherapy. *Semin. Immunol.* **22,** 183–189.

Peng, X., Hussain, S. F., and Paterson, Y. (2004). The ability of two Listeria monocytogenes vaccines targeting human papillomavirus-16 E7 to induce an antitumor response correlates with myeloid dendritic cell function. *J. Immunol.* **172,** 6030–6038.

Peng, X., Treml, J., and Paterson, Y. (2007). Adjuvant properties of listeriolysin O protein in a DNA vaccine strategy. *Cancer Immunol. Immunother.* **56,** 797–806.

Perez-Gomez, E., Villa-Morales, M., Santos, J., Fernandez-Piqueras, J., Gamallo, C., Dotor, J., Bernabeau, C., and Quintanilla, M. (2007). A role for endoglin as a suppressor of malignancy during mouse skin carcinogenesis. *Cancer Res.* **67,** 10268–10277.

Peters, C., and Paterson, Y. (2003). Enhancing the immunogenicity of bioengineered *Listeria monocytogenes* by passaging through live animal hosts. *Vaccine* **21,** 1187–1194.

Piccirillo, C. A., and Shevach, E. M. (2001). Cutting edge: Control of CD8(+) T cell activation by CD4(+)CD25(+) immunoregulatory cells. *J. Immunol.* **167,** 1137–1140.

Radford, K. J., Higgins, D. E., Pasquini, S., Cheadle, E. J., Carta, L., Jackson, A. M., Lemoine, N. R., and Vassaux, G. (2002). A recombinant *E. coli* vaccine to promote MHC class I-dependent antigen presentation: Application to cancer immunotherapy. *Gene Ther.* **9,** 1455–1463.

Read, S., Malmstrom, V., and Powrie, F. (2000). Cytotoxic T lymphocyte-associated antigen 4 plays an essential role in the function of CD25(+)CD4(+) regulatory cells that control intestinal inflammation. *J. Exp. Med.* **192,** 295–302.

Sakaguchi, S., Sakaguchi, N., Asano, M., Itoh, M., and Toda, M. (1995). Immunologic self-tolerance maintained by activated T cells expressing IL-2 receptor alpha-chains (CD25). Breakdown of a single mechanism of self-tolerance causes various autoimmune diseases. *J. Immunol.* **155,** 1151–1164.

Schafer, R., Portnoy, D. A., Brassell, S. A., and Paterson, Y. (1992). Induction of a cellular immune response to a foreign antigen by a recombinant *Listeria monocytogenes* vaccine. *J. Immunol.* **149,** 53–59.

Scheffner, M., Werness, B. A., Huibregtse, J. M., Levine, A. J., and Howley, P. M. (1990). The E6 oncoprotein encoded by human papillomavirus types 16 and 18 promotes the degradation of p53. *Cell* **63,** 1129–1136.

Schnupf, P., Hofmann, J., Norseen, J., Glomski, I. J., Schwartzstein, H., and Decatur, A. L. (2006). Regulated translation of listeriolysin O controls virulence of Listeria monocytogenes. *Mol. Microbiol.* **61,** 999–1012.

Schoen, C., Loeffler, D. I., Frentzen, A., Pilgrim, S., Goebel, W., and Stritzker, J. (2008). *Listeria monocytogenes* as novel carrier system for the development of live vaccines. *Int. J. Med. Microbiol.* **298,** 45–58.

Seavey, M. M., and Paterson, Y. (2009). Anti-angiogenesis immunotherapy induces epitope spreading to Her-2/neu resulting in tumor immunoediting. *Breast Cancer* **1,** 19–30.

Seavey, M. M., Verch, T., and Paterson, Y. (2008). Anticancer vaccine strategies. *In* "Handbook of *Listeria monocytogenes*", (D. Liu, ed.), pp. 481–511. CRC Press, USA.

Seavey, M. M., Pan, Z. K., Maciag, P. C., Wallecha, A., Rivera, S., Paterson, Y., and Shahabi, V. (2009a). A novel human Her-2/neu chimeric molecule expressed by *Listeria monocytogenes* can elicit potent HLA-A2 restricted CD8-positive T cell responses and impact the growth and spread of Her-2/neu-positive breast tumors. *Clin. Cancer Res.* **15,** 924–932.

Seavey, M. M., Pan, Z. K., Maciag, P. C., Wallecha, A., Rivera, S., Paterson, Y., and Shahabi, V. (2009b). An anti-vascular endothelial growth factor receptor 2/fetal liver kinase-1 *Listeria monocytogenes* anti-angiogenesis cancer vaccine for the treatment of primary and metastatic Her-2/neu+ breast tumors in a mouse model. *J. Immunol.* **182,** 5537–5546.

Seedorf, K., Oltersdorf, T., Krämmer, G., and Röwekamp, W. (1987). Identification of early proteins of the human papilloma viruses type 16 (HPV 16) and type 18 (HPV 18) in cervical carcinoma cells. *EMBO J.* **6,** 139–144.

Sewell, D. A., Douven, D., Pan, Z. K., Rodriguez, A., and Paterson, Y. (2004a). Regression of HPV-positive tumors treated with a new Listeria monocytogenes vaccine. *Arch. Otolaryngol. Head Neck Surg.* **130,** 92–97.

Sewell, D. A., Shahabi, V., Gunn, G. R., 3rd, Pan, Z. K., Dominiecki, M. E., and Paterson, Y. (2004b). Recombinant *Listeria* vaccines containing PEST sequences are potent immune adjuvants for the tumor-associated antigen human papillomavirus-16 E7. *Cancer Res.* **64,** 8821–8825.

Sewell, D. A., Pan, Z. K., and Paterson, Y. (2008). Listeria-based HPV-16 E7 vaccines limit autochthonous tumor growth in a transgenic mouse model for HPV-16 transformed tumors. *Vaccine* **26,** 5315–5320.

Shahabi, V., Reyes-Reyes, M., Wallecha, A., Rivera, S., Paterson, Y., and Maciag, P. C. (2008). Development of a Listeria monocytogenes based vaccine against prostate cancer. *Cancer Immunol. Immunother.* **57,** 1301–1313.

Shahabi, V., Seavey, M. M., Maciag, P. C., Rivera, S., and Wallecha, A. (2011). Development of a live and highly attenuated Listeria monocytogenes-based vaccine for the treatment of Her2/neu-overexpressing cancers in human. *Cancer Gene Ther.* **8,** 53–62.

Shibuya, M. (2006). Vascular endothelial growth factor (VEGF)-Receptor2, its biological functions, major signaling pathway, and specific ligand VEGF-E. *Endothelium* **13,** 63–69.

Singh, R., and Paterson, Y. (2006). Vaccination strategy determines the emergence and dominance of $CD8^+$ T-cell epitopes in a FVB/N rat HER-2/neu mouse model of breast cancer. *Cancer Res.* **66,** 7748–7757.

Singh, R., and Paterson, Y. (2007). Immunoediting sculpts tumor epitopes during immunotherapy. *Cancer Res.* **67,** 1887–1892.

Singh, R., Dominiecki, M. E., Jaffee, E. M., and Paterson, Y. (2005). Fusion to listeriolysin O and delivery by *Listeria monocytogenes* enhances the immunogenicity of HER-2/neu and reveals subdominant epitopes in the FVB/N mouse. *J. Immunol.* **175,** 3663–3673.

Souders, N. C., Verch, T., and Paterson, Y. (2006). In vivo bactofection, Listeria can function as a DNA-cancer vaccine. *DNA Cell Biol.* **25,** 142–151.

Souders, N. C., Sewell, D. A., Pan, Z. K., Hussain, S. F., Rodriguez, A., Wallecha, A., and Paterson, Y. (2007). Listeria-based vaccines can partially overcome tolerance by expanding low avidity CD8+ T cells capable of eradicating a solid tumor in a transgenic mouse model of cancer. *Cancer Immun.* **7,** 2.

Spreng, S., Gentschev, I., Goebel, W., Mollenkopf, H., Eck, M., Müller-Hermelink, H. K., and Schmausser, B. (2000). Novel bacterial systems for the delivery of recombinant protein or DNA. *FEMS Immunol. Med. Microbiol.* **27,** 299–304.

Starks, H., Bruhn, K. W., Shen, H., Barry, R. A., Dubensky, T. W., Brockstedt, D., Hinrichs, D. J., Higgins, D. E., Miller, J. F., Giedlin, M., and Bouwer, H. G. (2004). *Listeria monocytogenes* as a vaccine vector, virulence attenuation or existing antivector immunity does not diminish therapeutic efficacy. *J. Immunol.* **173,** 420–427.

Stritzker, J., Pilgrim, S., Szalay, A. A., and Goebel, W. (2008). Prodrug converting enzyme gene delivery by L. monocytogenes. *BMC Cancer* **8,** 94.

Takahashi, N., Kawanishi-Tabata, R., Haba, A., Tabata, M., Haruta, Y., Tsai, H., and Seon, B. K. (2001). Association of serum endoglin with metastasis in patients with colorectal, breast, and other solid tumors, and suppressive effect of chemotherapy on the serum endoglin. *Clin. Cancer Res.* **7,** 524–532.

Tam, M. A., and Wick, M. J. (2006). Differential expansion, activation and effector functions of conventional and plasmacytoid dendritic cells in mouse tissues transiently infected with Listeria monocytogenes. *Cell. Microbiol.* **8,** 1172–1187.

Tindle, R. W. (1996). Human papillomavirus vaccines for cervical cancer. *Curr. Opin. Immunol.* **8,** 643–650.

Tindle, R. W., and Frazer, I. H. (1994). Immune response to human papillomaviruses and the prospects for human papillomavirus-specific immunization. *Curr. Top. Microbiol. Immunol.* **186,** 217–253.

Torre-Amione, G., Beauchamp, R. D., Koeppen, H., Park, B. H., Schreiber, H., Moses, H. L., and Rowley, D. A. (1990). A highly immunogenic tumor transfected with a murine transforming growth factor type beta 1 cDNA escapes immune surveillance. *Proc. Natl. Acad. Sci. USA* **87,** 1486–1490.

Van den Eynde, B., Hainaut, P., Hérin, M., Knuth, A., Lemoine, C., Weynants, P., van der Bruggen, P., Fauchet, R., and Boon, T. (1989). Presence on a human melanoma of multiple antigens recognized by autologous CTL. *Int. J. Cancer* **44,** 634–640.

Velge, P., Bottreau, E., Kaeffer, B., and Pardon, P. (1994). Cell immortalization enhances Listeria monocytogenes invasion. *Med. Microbiol. Immunol.* **183,** 145–158.

Verch, T., Pan, Z. K., and Paterson, Y. (2004). *Listeria monocytogenes*-based antibiotic resistance gene-free antigen delivery system applicable to other bacterial vectors and DNA vaccines. *Infect. Immun.* **72,** 6418–6425.

Wadsworth, S., and Goldfine, H. (2002). Mobilization of proteinase C in macrophages induced by *Listeria monocytogenes* affects its internalization and escape from the phagosome. *Infect. Immun.* **70,** 4650–4660.

Wallecha, A., Carroll, K. D., Maciag, P. C., Rivera, S., Shahabi, V., and Paterson, Y. (2009a). Multiple effector mechanisms induced by recombinant *Listeria monocytogenes* anti-cancer immunotherapeutics. *Adv. Appl. Microbiol.* **66,** 1–27.

Wallecha, A., Maciag, P. C., Rivera, S., Paterson, Y., and Shahabi, V. (2009b). Construction and characterization of an attenuated *Listeria monocytogenes* strain for clinical use in cancer immunotherapy. *Clin. Vaccine Immunol.* **16,** 96–103.

Wang, J. M., Kumar, S., Pye, D., van Agthoven, A. J., Krupinski, J., and Hunter, R. D. (1993). A monoclonal antibody detects heterogeneity in vascular endothelium of tumours and normal tissues. *Int. J. Cancer* **54,** 363–370.

Weiskirch, L. M., and Paterson, Y. (1997). *Listeria monocytogenes,* a potent vaccine vector for neoplastic and infectious disease. *Immunol. Rev.* **158,** 159–169.

Wolf, S. F., Sieburth, D., and Sypek, J. (1994). Interleukin 12, a key modulator of immune function. *Stem Cells* **12,** 154–168.

Wood, L. M., Pan, Z. K., Shahabi, V., and Paterson, Y. (2010). Listeria-derived ActA is an effective adjuvant for primary and metastatic tumor immunotherapy. *Cancer Immunol. Immunother.* **59,** 1049–1058.

Wood, L. M., Pan, Z. K., Guirnalda, P., Tsai, P., Seavey, M. M., and Paterson, Y. (2011a). Targeting tumor vasculature with novel listeria-based vaccines directed against CD105. *Cancer Immunol. Immunother.* **60,** 931–942.

Wood, L. M., Seavey, M. M., Pan, Z. K., and Paterson, Y. (2011b). Targeting the tumor-associated ubiquitin-like protein, ISG15, as a novel strategy for breast cancer treatment. *Cancer Immunol. Immunother.* In Press.

Yu, Y. A., Shabahang, S., Timiryasova, T. M., Zhang, Q., Beltz, R., Gentschev, I., Goebel, W., and Szalay, A. A. (2004). Visualization of tumors and metastases in live animals with bacteria and vaccinia virus encoding light-emitting proteins. *Nat. Biotechnol.* **22,** 313–320.

CHAPTER 7

Monocyte-Mediated Immune Defense Against Murine *Listeria monocytogenes* Infection

Natalya V. Serbina, Chao Shi, and **Eric G. Pamer**

Contents

Infectious Diseases Service, Department of Medicine, Immunology Program, Sloan-Kettering Institute, Memorial Sloan-Kettering Cancer Center, New York, USA

Advances in Immunology, Volume 113
ISSN 0065-2776, DOI: 10.1016/B978-0-12-394590-7.00003-8

Abstract

Infection of mice with *Listeria monocytogenes* induces a robust innate inflammatory response that restricts bacterial growth in the liver and spleen prior to the development of protective T cell responses. Ly6C^{hi} monocytes contribute to the innate immune response following *L. monocytogenes* infection and in their absence, mice rapidly succumb to infection. Emigration of Ly6C^{hi} monocytes from the bone marrow into the circulation is the first step in their recruitment to sites of *L. monocytogenes* infection and is triggered by CCL2- and CCL7-mediated stimulation of CCR2 chemokine receptors on monocytes. CCL2 expression by mesenchymal stem cells in the bone marrow, in response to TLR stimulation, drives monocyte emigration from cellular compartments into vascular sinuses of the bone marrow. In addition to TLR ligands, type I interferon-mediated signals can also drive monocyte emigration from the bone marrow during *L. monocytogenes* infection. Once Ly6C^{hi} monocytes enter the bloodstream, trafficking to sites of infection in the liver and spleen is CCR2 independent. In the liver, CD11b on the monocyte and ICAM-1 on the surface of endothelial cells target Ly6C^{hi} monocytes to foci of *L. monocytogenes* infection. At the site of infection, Ly6C^{hi} monocytes undergo MyD88-dependent differentiation into TNF and iNOS-producing dendritic cells (TipDCs) and express MHC class II, B7.1, and CD40 on their cell surface. How TipDCs mediate bacterial clearance during early *L. monocytogenes* infection remains an active area of investigation.

1. MONOCYTES AND THE DISCOVERY OF *LISTERIA MONOCYTOGENES*

A potentially important role for monocytes in defense against *L. monocytogenes* infection was suggested as early as 1926 when investigators from Cambridge University described a lethal infection of rabbits that was caused by a previously unknown Gram-positive bacterium. Because these rabbits developed a marked monocytosis, the organism was named *Bacterium monocytogenes* (Murray *et al.*, 1926). A report the following year described a lethal infection of gerbils in South Africa, again caused by an unknown Gram-positive bacterium. This organism was named *Listerella hepatolytica; Listerella* in honor of Sir Joseph Lister (who had died 15 years earlier) and *hepatolytica* because this bacterium caused hepatic necrosis (Pirie, 1927). Subsequent studies determined that *B. monocytogenes* and *L. hepatolytica* are the same organism and bacterial taxonomists eventually settled on the name *L. monocytogenes*. Another 60 years passed before the role of monocytes in defense against *L. monocytogenes* infection was more completely characterized.

2. MONOCYTE POPULATIONS CIRCULATING IN THE MOUSE BLOODSTREAM

The past 5 years have seen great advances in our understanding of circulating monocytes, a subset of blood leukocytes that until recently received far less attention than other circulating white blood cells (Auffray *et al.*, 2009a,b). In mice, chemokine receptor expression has been used to distinguish distinct monocyte subsets that differ in terms of trafficking under homeostatic and inflammatory/infectious conditions (Geissmann *et al.*, 2003; Palframan *et al.*, 2001). One subset of circulating monocytes expresses the Ly6C surface marker and the CCR2 chemokine receptor. This subset traffics to sites of inflammation and infection, and these cells are therefore often referred to as inflammatory or Ly6C^{hi} monocytes (Auffray *et al.*, 2009a,b). A second subset of murine monocytes is distinguished by high expression of the CX3CR1 chemokine receptor and low Ly6C expression (Geissmann *et al.*, 2003). These cells, referred to as CX3CR1^{hi} or Ly6C^{lo} monocytes, have distinct trafficking characteristics, which include LFA-1-dependent patrolling on the luminal surface of small blood vessels (Auffray *et al.*, 2007). Their role in defense against infectious diseases is less well defined, although they have been implicated in very early responses to *L. monocytogenes* infection (Auffray *et al.*, 2009a,b).

3. CCR2-MEDIATED MONOCYTE RECRUITMENT

Inflammatory monocyte recruitment to sites of infection is mediated by CCR2 on the monocyte, and the chemokines CC-chemokine ligand 2 (CCL2, also referred to as MCP1) and CCL7 (also known as MCP3) (Tsou *et al.*, 2007). Many nucleated cells can express CCL2 in response to a range of stimuli (Brown *et al.*, 1994; Rollins and Pober, 1991; Struyf *et al.*, 1998; Tsou *et al.*, 2007; Tsuboi *et al.*, 2002). The dramatic induction of CCL2 expression during infection, in part triggered by stimulation of TLRs by microbial molecules (Tsuboi *et al.*, 2002), suggested that CCR2-expressing monocytes follow a gradient of CCL2 from the bloodstream to the infected focus. CCL2, like many chemokines, is known to dimerize and associate with glycosaminoglycans (GAGs), and some experimental evidence supports the notion that association with GAGs is required for CCL2's *in vivo* activity (Allen *et al.*, 2007; Proudfoot *et al.*, 2003). Although much less studied, CCL7 also contributes to Ly6C^{hi} monocyte recruitment (Jia *et al.*, 2008; Tsou *et al.*, 2007) and will be discussed in greater detail in later sections. While chemokines are believed to provide monocytes with a sense of direction during their recruitment, the mechanics of recruitment are mediated by integrins and other adhesion molecules (Ley *et al.*, 2007).

4. MYELOID CELLS IN DEFENSE AGAINST *L. MONOCYTOGENES*

The importance of myeloid cells in defense against *L. monocytogenes* infection was first demonstrated by Rosen and colleagues, in studies using the 5C6 monoclonal antibody, which blocks CD11b and thus prevents inflammatory cell trafficking into infected tissues. In this study, administration of this blocking antibody at the initiation of infection resulted in uncontrolled growth of *L. monocytogenes* in the livers of infected mice, while blockade at later stages of infection was far less immunocompromising (Rosen *et al.*, 1989). Histologic examination of the livers of 5C6-treated mice following infection demonstrated markedly reduced myeloid cell infiltration and far greater hepatic necrosis and bacterial growth, leading the investigators to conclude that these myeloid cells restrict infection of hepatocytes. This study, however, could not distinguish between monocytes and neutrophils, as trafficking of both of these populations was inhibited by CD11b blockade. A subsequent study by Kurihara and colleagues investigated *L. monocytogenes* infection of mice genetically engineered to lack the CCR2 chemokine receptor (Kurihara *et al.*, 1997). Systemic infection of CCR2-deficient mice with *L. monocytogenes* demonstrated their marked susceptibility, with greatly reduced clearance of bacteria from the spleen and liver and far greater hepatic necrosis. These authors recognized that CCR2 deficiency resulted in reduced recruitment of mononuclear phagocytes to sites of infection and demonstrated the importance of this cell population and this chemokine receptor in defense against *L. monocytogenes*.

5. LY6C^{HI} MONOCYTES AND TIPDCS DURING *L. MONOCYTOGENES* INFECTION

Although the roles of CCR2 and CD11b in defense against *L. monocytogenes* were well established by these studies, the cells that mediate antibacterial defense during the early stages of infection remained incompletely defined. To begin a characterization of monocyte-mediated antimicrobial defense, wild-type and CCR2-deficient mice were infected with *L. monocytogenes* and inflammatory cell recruitment to the spleen over the first 3 days of infection was investigated (Serbina *et al.*, 2003b). These studies demonstrated that *L. monocytogenes* infection resulted in the recruitment of CD11b and Mac-3 expressing cells in wild-type mice and that the frequency of these cells was markedly reduced in CCR2-deficient mice. CD11b$^+$Mac-3$^+$ cells also expressed low levels of CD11c and morphologically resembled dendritic cells. Further characterization of these cells demonstrated that they produced high levels of TNF and iNOS and expressed CD40, B7.1, B7.2, and high levels of MHC class II on the cell surface. Because these cells were able to prime naïve alloreactive T cells and produced TNF and iNOS, they were named TNF/iNOS-producing dendritic cells (TipDCs). A remarkable characteristic of these cells is that they were recruited to foci of *L. monocytogenes* infection in the white pulp of the spleen and, although not directly infected, were the major producers of TNF and iNOS. Thus, in CCR2-deficient mice, splenic TNF and iNOS levels were markedly reduced following *L. monocytogenes* infection. As both TNF and iNOS had been demonstrated in previous studies to be essential for clearance of murine *L. monocytogenes* infection (MacMicking *et al.*, 1995; Pfeffer *et al.*, 1993; Rothe *et al.*, 1993), the identification of TipDCs as their source provided new insight into cellular mechanisms of antimicrobial defense. Further, the finding that TNF and iNOS are predominantly produced by cells that do not harbor live bacteria suggested that stimuli from infected cells and the release of microbial products from foci of infection drive the production of these critical immune mediators. The ability of CCR2-expressing monocytes to confer resistance to *L. monocytogenes* infection was demonstrated by their adoptive transfer into infected, CCR2-deficient recipient mice. In these experiments, adoptive transfer of CCR2-expressing monocytes enhanced bacterial clearance from the spleen (Serbina *et al.*, 2003b).

6. THE ROLE OF CCL2 AND CCL7 IN MONOCYTE RECRUITMENT

Recruitment of TipDCs to the spleen was CCR2 dependent, suggesting that *L. monocytogenes* infection induced the expression of CCR2 ligands, such as CCL2. Indeed, earlier studies had demonstrated that *L. monocytogenes* infection is accompanied by *in vivo* expression of chemokines, including CCL2 (Barsig *et al.*, 1998). *In vivo* production of CCL2, however, required inoculation of mice with strains of *L. monocytogenes* that gain access to the host cell cytosol (Serbina *et al.*, 2003a). Thus, infection of mice with strains of *L. monocytogenes* that lacked listeriolysin-O, the essential virulence factor that enables bacteria to escape the vacuole and enter the cytosol, did not induce detectable levels of CCL2 expression in the spleen. Similarly, inoculation of mice with heat-killed *L. monocytogenes* also did not induce CCL2 expression. However, infection of mice with an attenuated strain of *L. monocytogenes* lacking ActA, a virulence factor that facilitates actin polymerization and intracytoplasmic motility, induced *in vivo* CCL2 expression. ActA-deficient *L. monocytogenes*, though attenuated, accesses the cytoplasm of host cells, suggesting that this step is essential for induction of CCL2 during *in vivo* infection. Consistent with this result, TipDC recruitment to the spleen is normal in mice inoculated with ActA-deficient *L. monocytogenes,* while neither LLO-deficient nor heat-killed *L. monocytogenes* administration resulted in TipDC recruitment to the spleen.

To determine whether CCL2 contributes to defense against *L. monocytogenes* infection, CCL2-deficient mice were infected and the course of infection was monitored. These studies demonstrated that CCL2 contributes to bacterial clearance, although CCL2-deficient mice are not as sensitive to *L. monocytogenes* infection as CCR2-deficient mice. TipDC recruitment to the spleen of CCL2-deficient mice is reduced by approximately 60%, suggesting that the intermediate phenotype of CCL2-deficient as opposed to CCR2-deficient mice results from reduced but not absent recruitment of this cell population to sites of infection (Serbina *et al.*, 2003a). This result also suggested that other chemokines can stimulate CCR2-mediated Ly6C^{hi} monocyte recruitment during *L. monocytogenes* infection.

To address this possibility, CCL7-deficient mice were investigated. CCR2 also responds to stimulation by CCL7, and mice deficient for CCL7 have diminished recruitment of Ly6C^{hi} monocytes to sites of inflammation (Tsou *et al.*, 2007). Murine infection with *L. monocytogenes* induces CCL7 expression in serum, blood, liver, and kidney with kinetics that are similar to CCL2 expression (Jia *et al.*, 2008). Tissue levels of CCL7 and CCL2 differ, however, with the amount of CCL7 exceeding the amount of CCL2 in the kidneys of infected mice. Peak chemokine concentrations are present in these tissues approximately 48 h after intravenous infection, correlating with the peak of bacterial infection. Similar to CCL2 induction by *L. monocytogenes* infection, only cytoplasm invasive strains of *L. monocytogenes* induce *in vivo* expression of CCL7. Thus, inoculation of mice with LLO-deficient and heat-killed bacteria did not induce CCL7 expression. Along similar lines, tissue culture bone marrow macrophages produce CCL7 in response to virulent *L. monocytogenes* infection, but induction of CCL7 is markedly reduced in response to LLO-deficient or heat-killed bacteria (Jia *et al.*, 2008). CCL7-deficient mice are more susceptible to *L. monocytogenes* infection. Similar to CCL2-deficient mice, mice lacking CCL7 are not as susceptible as CCR2-deficient mice, but they are more susceptible than wild-type mice. Infection of mice lacking CCL7 with virulent *L. monocytogenes* results in approximately 50% reduced recruitment of TipDCs to infected spleens when compared to infected wild-type mice. These results suggest that CCL2 and CCL7 make nonredundant contributions to CCR2-dependent recruitment of monocytes to sites of *L. monocytogenes* infection. It remains unclear, however, whether CCL2 and CCL7 contributions in wild-type mice are simply additive or whether these two chemokines function in physically distinct sites during infection.

7. CCL2 EXPRESSION DURING *L. MONOCYTOGENES* INFECTION

To begin to determine the upstream signaling pathways that trigger CCL2 expression in response to *L. monocytogenes* infection, MyD88-, TNF-, and Caspase-1-deficient mice were infected and chemokine levels were measured in the spleen. In comparison to wild-type mice, CCL2 expression in the infected spleens was modestly decreased in TNF-, Caspase-1 (and therefore IL-1)-, and MyD88-deficient mice (Serbina *et al.*, 2003a). MyD88 deficiency had been shown previously to markedly increase susceptibility to *L. monocytogenes* infection (Edelson and Unanue, 2002; Seki *et al.*, 2002). Recruitment of inflammatory monocytes to the spleen of MyD88-deficient mice following *L. monocytogenes* inoculation was not reduced during the first 2 days of infection. However, production of TNF and iNOS by recruited monocytes in the spleen of infected mice was markedly reduced. This study, therefore, demonstrated that monocyte recruitment, during the first 2–3 days following infection, is driven by a MyD88-independent, innate immune signaling pathway that is triggered by bacterial invasion of the host cell's cytoplasm. Differentiation of recruited monocytes into TipDCs, however, is MyD88 dependent and likely occurs as a result of TLR-mediated signals in response to microbial molecules at the site of infection (Serbina *et al.*, 2003a). *L. monocytogenes* infection induces splenic dendritic cells to recruit and cluster NK cells and inflammatory monocytes at sites of infection, and interferon-γ produced by NK cells contributes to MyD88-dependent differentiation of Ly6C^{hi} monocytes into TipDCs (Kang *et al.*, 2008).

8. *L. MONOCYTOGENES* INFECTION INCREASES MONOCYTOPOIESIS

Recruitment of neutrophils and monocytes to peripheral sites is essential for defense against a number of microbial pathogens. Under homeostatic conditions, the frequency of these cells in peripheral tissues is low. Following infection, their numbers increase due, in part, to accelerated emigration from bone marrow and, in part, to enhanced recruitment into inflamed tissues. Although recruitment and activation of myeloid cells in peripheral tissues have been studied, relatively little is known about inflammation-driven bone marrow hematopoiesis. In order to address this issue, bone marrow myeloid populations were characterized following infection with *L. monocytogenes* (Serbina *et al.*, 2009). These studies demonstrated that inflammation induced by *L. monocytogenes* infection dramatically changes the hematopoietic compartment of the bone marrow and specifically promotes monopoiesis. In contrast to the effect of infection on monocyte production, granulocyte production in the bone marrow was decreased during later stages of infection and, accordingly, monocytes and not granulocytes were increasingly recruited to infected spleen as infection progressed. In the absence of Myd88/Trif-mediated signaling, monocyte frequencies and proliferation of monocyte precursors were diminished in the bone marrow beyond 72 h of *L. monocytogenes* infection. This study demonstrated that proliferation and replenishment of monocyte precursors are dependant on ongoing inflammation and require TLR-mediated signaling. Thus, innate immune deficiency resulting from loss of Myd88 expression stems not only from inadequate cell activation during infection but also from the inability to replenish innate immune effector cells, in particular, Ly6C^{hi} monocytes.

9. TYPE I INTERFERON EFFECTS ON CCL2 EXPRESSION

Infection of host cells by cytosol invasive *L. monocytogenes* results in the expression of type I interferon (O'Riordan *et al.*, 2002). Interferon-β and interferons-α signal via the type I interferon receptor (IFNAR), and type I interferon signaling is abolished in IFNAR-deficient mice. While type I interferon signaling is deleterious during *L. monocytogenes* infection (Auerbuch *et al.*, 2004; Carrero *et al.*, 2004; O'Connell *et al.*, 2004), this signaling pathway is capable of stimulating CCL2 expression (Hokeness-Antonelli *et al.*, 2007). To determine the relative contributions of MyD88 and IFNAR to the induction of CCL2 expression during *L. monocytogenes* infection, MyD88, IFNAR, and MyD88/IFNAR double-deficient mice were infected and CCL2 levels were measured in the spleen and serum (Jia *et al.*, 2009). These studies demonstrated that combined deletion of MyD88 and IFNAR signaling markedly reduced CCL2 production.

Analysis of bone marrow macrophages demonstrated that MyD88-mediated signals induced CCL2 mRNA within 30 min of infection and that IFNAR-mediated signals amplified CCL2 mRNA levels between 1 and 6 h after infection. Ly6C^{hi} monocyte recruitment to spleens following *L. monocytogenes* infection was normal in IFNAR- and MyD88-deficient mice but was markedly reduced in mice with combined deficiency of IFNAR and MyD88. Thus, with respect to monocyte recruitment during *L. monocytogenes* infection, IFNAR and MyD88 signaling pathways provide some redundancy that ensures monocyte recruitment.

While MyD88-deficient mice are highly susceptible to *L. monocytogenes* infection, and IFNAR-deficient mice are more resistant, double-deficient mice are even more susceptible to infection than MyD88-deficient mice. This result suggests that type I interferon-mediated signals can be protective, but only in the absence of TLR signaling. Previous studies had demonstrated that *L. monocytogenes* infection induces T cell apoptosis in the white pulp of the spleen, inducing IL-10 production and downregulating innate immune defenses (Carrero *et al.*, 2004; Tripp *et al.*, 1993). Type I interferon induction during infection enhances T cell apoptosis and thus enhances IL10 production (Carrero *et al.*, 2004, 2006), thereby reducing innate immune resistance to *L. monocytogenes* infection. In IFNAR-deficient mice, T cell apoptosis following *L. monocytogenes* infection is reduced, thereby paradoxically enhancing resistance because IL-10 expression is presumably decreased. If IL-10 induction during *L. monocytogenes* infection is MyD88 dependent, then the immunocompromising effect of type I interferon expression would be negated by MyD88 deficiency. Thus, by eliminating the immunocompromising effect, MyD88 deficiency reveals the protective effect of type I interferon signaling.

10. CCR2-DEFICIENT LY6C^{HI} MONOCYTES ARE RETAINED IN THE BONE MARROW

Recruitment of Ly6C^{hi} monocytes during *L. monocytogenes* infection is a multistep process that culminates in the arrival of TipDCs at sites of infection. Although it seemed likely that CCR2 would mediate the recruitment of circulating Ly6C^{hi} monocytes from the bloodstream to infected tissues, careful analysis of bloodstream monocyte frequencies in *L. monocytogenes*-infected, CCR2-deficient mice revealed a marked paucity of monocytes in the blood (Serbina and Pamer, 2006). Even more surprising, frequencies of Ly6C^{hi} monocytes in the blood of uninfected CCR2-deficient mice were also markedly reduced compared to uninfected wild-type mice, suggesting that homeostatic regulation of Ly6C^{hi} monocyte frequencies is CCR2 dependent. Further analysis revealed that Ly6C^{hi} monocyte frequencies were increased in the bone marrow of CCR2-deficient mice and, in the setting of *L. monocytogenes* infection, the frequency of these cells markedly increased and they upregulated MHC class II and B7.1 expression and produced TNF in the bone marrow. In contrast to Ly6C^{hi} monocytes that trafficked to the spleen in wild-type mice, Ly6C^{hi} monocytes that were retained in the bone marrow of *L. monocytogenes*-infected, CCR2-deficient mice did not express iNOS or upregulate the expression of CD11c. The reason for this disparity is unknown, but it may be the result of diminished exposure of bone marrow-retained monocytes to bacterially derived TLR ligands, which drive TipDC differentiation in the spleen. Although to a lesser extent than in CCR2-deficient mice, CCL2 deficiency also resulted in decreased emigration of Ly6C^{hi} monocytes from the bone marrow into the bloodstream (Serbina and Pamer, 2006). CCL7 also contributes to homeostatic monocyte emigration from the bone marrow. The frequency of Ly6C^{hi} monocytes in the circulation of CCL7-deficient mice is reduced by approximately 60%, while the frequency of monocytes in the bone marrow is increased. During *L. monocytogenes* infection of CCL7-deficient mice, the frequency of Ly6C^{hi} monocytes in the bone marrow remained elevated, a result of diminished emigration into the bloodstream (Jia *et al.*, 2008).

11. Ly6C^{HI} MONOCYTE RECRUITMENT TO INFECTED TISSUES

Although CCR2-signaling mediates monocyte emigration from the bone marrow into the bloodstream, whether CCR2 also contributes to tissue infiltration by Ly6C^{hi} monocytes remains more controversial. To determine whether CCR2 is required for Ly6C^{hi} monocyte recruitment from the bloodstream into the spleens of *L. monocytogenes*-infected mice, blood monocytes from CCR2-deficient or CCR2-sufficient mice were transferred into infected recipient mice and their trafficking to the spleen was quantified (Serbina and Pamer, 2006). *L. monocytogenes* infection in spleen is largely restricted to the T cell zones of the white pulp (Conlan, 1996), so localization of monocytes to infected white pulp regions was also measured. These studies demonstrated that localization of CCR2-deficient and -sufficient monocytes in the spleen was similar, suggesting that CCR2 is not required for trafficking from the bloodstream into the spleen or, within the spleen, into foci of *L. monocytogenes* infection within the white pulp.

Infection of the liver is also markedly enhanced in CCR2-deficient mice (Kurihara *et al.*, 1997). Ly6C^{hi} monocytes are infrequent in uninfected livers, representing only 1–2% of CD45^{+} cells, but, upon *L. monocytogenes* infection, their frequency increases dramatically, and they represent nearly 30% of CD45^{+} cells 3 days following intravenous inoculation (Shi *et al.*, 2010). Histologic analyses demonstrated that Ly6C^{hi} monocytes localize to sites of *L. monocytogenes* infection in the liver, surrounding foci of bacteria and necrotic hepatocytes. Monocytes recruited to the liver express TNF and iNOS and upregulate surface MHC class II expression and thus are similar to splenic TipDCs. Adoptive transfer of wild-type or CCR2-deficient monocytes into *L. monocytogenes*-infected recipient mice demonstrated that they trafficked similarly to foci of infection in the liver. Intravital microscopy demonstrated that the velocity and arrest and meandering indices of CCR2-deficient and CCR2-sufficient Ly6C^{hi} monocytes were similar in the livers of infected mice, suggesting that CCR2 does not contribute to monocyte recruitment or localization during hepatic *L. monocytogenes* infection.

Transfer of wild-type or CCR2-deficient monocytes into *L. monocytogenes*-infected, CCR2-deficient recipient mice protected against hepatic infection equivalently, demonstrating that CCR2-mediated signals are not required for intravenously inoculated monocytes to enter the liver and mediate protection. Treatment of adoptively transferred monocytes with pertussis toxin, which inhibits signaling by G-protein-coupled chemokine receptors, did not alter their trafficking to foci of *L. monocytogenes* infection in the liver, suggesting that monocyte recruitment from the bloodstream is not only CCR2 independent but generally chemokine independent (Shi *et al.*, 2010). Immunohistology demonstrated that hepatic foci of *L. monocytogenes* infected are surrounded by a zone of markedly upregulated ICAM-1 expression. ICAM-1 upregulation occurs on hepatic endothelial cells. Ly6C^{hi} monocytes localize to these sites of ICAM-1 upregulation in the liver, suggesting that monocytes are trapped in these areas. In support of this hypothesis, administration of blocking antibodies specific for ICAM-1, or CD11b, which binds ICAM-1, markedly reduces accumulation of Ly6C^{hi} monocytes in the liver (Shi *et al.*, 2010). These findings, in aggregate, suggest that monocytes localize to sites of infection in the liver by associating with ICAM-1 and that chemokine-mediated signals are not required for this process.

12. MONOCYTE EMIGRATION FROM THE BONE MARROW

Although the important role for CCR2 in the emigration of monocytes from the bone marrow has been demonstrated in many different infectious disease models (Aldridge *et al.*, 2009; Bosschaerts *et al.*, 2010; Crane *et al.*, 2009; Lim *et al.*, 2011), how infection in the lung, intestine, liver, or other central organs promotes monocyte emigration from bone marrow has been unclear. One possibility is that low-grade infection of the bone marrow serves as a stimulus to promote monocyte emigration from the bone marrow, a scenario for which there is little evidence and which seems counterintuitive (i.e., dispatching inflammatory cells away from a site of infection). Alternatively, systemic infections might induce local production of chemokines that enter the circulation and trigger responses in the bone marrow. This model is plausible but would require synthesis and secretion of large quantities of chemokine. Measurement of circulating chemokine levels reveals that they are produced in large quantities, but generally during late stages of infection. A third possibility is that the bone marrow detects low levels of circulating microbial molecules during infection and responds by expressing chemokines that promote inflammatory cell emigration into the bloodstream. This model would require the bone marrow compartment to detect circulating microbial molecules with great sensitivity, and it would require chemokines, CCL2 in the case of *L. monocytogenes* infection, to drive monocytes into the bloodstream.

To determine whether circulating microbial molecules influence bloodstream monocyte frequencies, TLR2, TLR4, TLR5, and TLR9 ligands were administered to mice and shown to markedly increase circulating Ly6C^{hi} inflammatory monocyte frequencies (Shi *et al.*, 2011). Increases in circulating monocyte frequencies in response to different TLR ligands required expression of the corresponding TLR. Thus, LPS administration did not induce monocyte emigration from the bone marrow in the absence of TLR4. Ly6C^{hi} monocyte frequencies in the bloodstream only increased when TLR ligands were administered at low concentrations. The dosage of LPS that increased the frequency of circulating monocytes ranged from 2 to 200 ng and higher doses of LPS did not increase circulating monocyte frequencies. The ineffectiveness of higher doses of LPS was surprising and may be the result of monocyte retention in the bone marrow by mechanisms that remain incompletely defined. In contrast to monocyte emigration from the bone marrow, neutrophils are recruited into the bloodstream by high doses of LPS.

Because many nucleated cells can produce CCL2 upon stimulation, it has remained unclear which CCL2-producing cells *in vivo* are driving monocyte trafficking. To determine whether CCL2 production by bone marrow-derived cell populations is required for monocyte trafficking, bone marrow chimeric mice were generated between CCL2-deficient and wild-type mice. These experiments demonstrated that CCL2 production by nonhematopoietic cells is required for monocyte emigration from the bone marrow (Shi *et al.*, 2011). This suggested that stromal cells, endothelial cells, or perhaps hepatocytes were producing CCL2 in order to drive monocyte emigration from the bone marrow into the bloodstream. To determine which cells produced CCL2 *in vivo* during *L. monocytogenes* infection, CCL2-reporter mice were generated. As a first step, BAC-transgenic mice in which the CCL2 promoter drives EGFP expression were produced. To simplify interpretation of this experiment, CCL2-EGFP reporter mice were irradiated and transplanted with wild-type bone marrow to restrict EGFP expression to nonhematopoietic cells. Infection of these mice with *L. monocytogenes*, or inoculation with low doses of LPS, demonstrated that CCL2 expression, as determined by EGFP fluorescence, was induced in stromal and endothelial cells of the bone marrow. Flow cytometric analysis revealed that the majority of CCL2-expressing cells were mesenchymal stem cells (MSCs) and/or CXCL12 abundant reticular (CAR) cells (Mendez-Ferrer *et al.*, 2010; Sugiyama *et al.*, 2006). These cells express TLR-2, -3, -4, -8, and -9 and reside in close proximity to bone marrow endothelial cells, and are also referred to as pericytes. These results suggested that MSCs and/or CAR cells respond to TLR ligands or to systemic *L. monocytogenes* infection and produce CCL2.

To determine whether CCL2 production by MSCs is required for monocyte emigration from the bone marrow, a conditional CCL2 knockout mouse strain was generated and crossed to the Nestin-Cre mouse (Shi *et al.*, 2011). Previous studies had demonstrated that bone marrow MSCs express Nestin (Mendez-Ferrer *et al.*, 2010), and thus, Nestin-Cre mice selectively delete CCL2 from MSCs in the bone marrow. Using this system, it was demonstrated that CCL2 production by MSCs contributes to monocyte emigration in response to low-dose administration of LPS and during *L. monocytogenes* infection. Further, deletion of CCL2 in MSCs renders mice more susceptible to *L. monocytogenes* infection, with decreased bacterial clearance from the liver and spleen. This study demonstrated that a stromal cell population monitors the circulation for the presence of microbial molecules and regulates the emigration of Ly6C^{hi} monocytes from the bone marrow in the bloodstream.

13. CONCLUSIONS

The past decade has seen great progress in our understanding of monocyte-mediated immune defense against viral and microbial pathogens (Serbina *et al.*, 2008); however, many questions remain unanswered. While inflammatory monocytes and their progeny, TipDCs, play an essential role in defense against *L. monocytogenes* infection, and the absence of Ly6C^{hi} monocytes renders mice highly susceptible, it remains unclear how monocytes mediate bacterial clearance in the liver and spleen. While TNF and iNOS contribute to innate immune defense, and TipDCs are the major producers of these two proteins during early infection, it is unknown whether TNF or iNOS production by TipDCs is essential for their antimicrobial activity. Questions about monocyte emigration from the bone marrow, such as how CCL2 and CCL7 mediate Ly6C^{hi} monocyte trafficking from the abluminal to luminal side of bone marrow endothelial cells, also remain unanswered. Given the increasing number of useful mouse strains that enable intravital analyses of monocyte trafficking, it is likely that our understanding of monocytes and their role in defense against murine *L. monocytogenes* infection will continue to increase in the coming years.

REFERENCES

Aldridge, J. R., Jr., Moseley, C. E., Boltz, D. A., Negovetich, N. J., Reynolds, C., Franks, J., Brown, S. A., Doherty, P. C., Webster, R. G., and Thomas, P. G. (2009). TNF/iNOS-producing dendritic cells are the necessary evil of lethal influenza virus infection. *Proc. Natl. Acad. Sci. USA* **106,** 5306.

Allen, S. J., Crown, S. E., and Handel, T. M. (2007). Chemokine: Receptor structure, interactions, and antagonism. *Annu. Rev. Immunol.* **25,** 787.

Auerbuch, V., Brockstedt, D. G., Meyer-Morse, N., O'Riordan, M., and Portnoy, D. A. (2004). Mice lacking the type I interferon receptor are resistant to Listeria monocytogenes. *J. Exp. Med.* **200,** 527.

Auffray, C., Fogg, D., Garfa, M., Elain, G., Join-Lambert, O., Kayal, S., Sarnacki, S., Cumano, A., Lauvau, G., and Geissmann, F. (2007). Monitoring of blood vessels and tissues by a population of monocytes with patrolling behavior. *Science* **317,** 666.

Auffray, C., Fogg, D. K., Narni-Mancinelli, E., Senechal, B., Trouillet, C., Saederup, N., Leemput, J., Bigot, K., Campisi, L., Abitbol, M., Molina, T., Charo, I., *et al.* (2009a). CX3CR1+ CD115+ CD135+ common macrophage/DC precursors and the role of CX3CR1 in their response to inflammation. *J. Exp. Med.* **206,** 595.

Auffray, C., Sieweke, M. H., and Geissmann, F. (2009b). Blood monocytes: Development, heterogeneity, and relationship with dendritic cells. *Annu. Rev. Immunol.* **27,** 669.

Barsig, J., Flesch, I. E., and Kaufmann, S. H. (1998). Macrophages and hepatocytic cells as chemokine producers in murine listeriosis. *Immunobiology* **199,** 87.

Bosschaerts, T., Guilliams, M., Stijlemans, B., Morias, Y., Engel, D., Tacke, F., Herin, M., De Baetselier, P., and Beschin, A. (2010). Tip-DC development during parasitic infection is regulated by IL-10 and requires CCL2/CCR2, IFN-gamma and MyD88 signaling. *PLoS Pathog.* **6,** e1001045.

Brown, Z., Gerritsen, M. E., Carley, W. W., Strieter, R. M., Kunkel, S. L., and Westwick, J. (1994). Chemokine gene expression and secretion by cytokine-activated human microvascular endothelial cells. Differential regulation of monocyte chemoattractant protein-1 and interleukin-8 in response to interferon-gamma. *Am. J. Pathol.* **145,** 913.

Carrero, J. A., Calderon, B., and Unanue, E. R. (2004). Type I interferon sensitizes lymphocytes to apoptosis and reduces resistance to listeria infection. *J. Exp. Med.* **200,** 535.

Carrero, J. A., Calderon, B., and Unanue, E. R. (2006). Lymphocytes are detrimental during the early innate immune response against Listeria monocytogenes. *J. Exp. Med.* **203,** 933.

Conlan, J. W. (1996). Early pathogenesis of Listeria monocytogenes infection in the mouse spleen. *J. Med. Microbiol.* **44,** 295.

Crane, M. J., Hokeness-Antonelli, K. L., and Salazar-Mather, T. P. (2009). Regulation of inflammatory monocyte/macrophage recruitment from the bone marrow during murine cytomegalovirus infection: Role for type I interferons in localized induction of CCR2 ligands. *J. Immunol.* **183,** 2810.

Edelson, B. T., and Unanue, E. R. (2002). MyD88-dependent but Toll-like receptor 2-independent innate immunity to Listeria: No role for either in macrophage listericidal activity. *J. Immunol.* **169,** 3869.

Geissmann, F., Jung, S., and Littman, D. R. (2003). Blood monocytes consist of two principal subsets with distinct migratory properties. *Immunity* **19,** 71.

Hokeness-Antonelli, K. L., Crane, M. J., Dragoi, A. M., Chu, W. M., and Salazar-Mather, T. P. (2007). IFN-alphabeta-mediated inflammatory responses and antiviral defense in liver is TLR9-independent but MyD88-dependent during murine cytomegalovirus infection. *J. Immunol.* **179,** 6176.

Jia, T., Serbina, N. V., Brandl, K., Zhong, M. X., Leiner, I. M., Charo, I. F., and Pamer, E. G. (2008). Additive roles for MCP-1 and MCP-3 in CCR2-mediated recruitment of inflammatory monocytes during Listeria monocytogenes infection. *J. Immunol.* **180,** 6846.

Jia, T., Leiner, I., Dorothee, G., Brandl, K., and Pamer, E. G. (2009). MyD88 and Type I interferon receptor-mediated chemokine induction and monocyte recruitment during Listeria monocytogenes infection. *J. Immunol.* **183,** 1271.

Kang, S. J., Liang, H. E., Reizis, B., and Locksley, R. M. (2008). Regulation of hierarchical clustering and activation of innate immune cells by dendritic cells. *Immunity* **29,** 819.

Kurihara, T., Warr, G., Loy, J., and Bravo, R. (1997). Defects in macrophage recruitment and host defense in mice lacking the CCR2 chemokine receptor. *J. Exp. Med.* **186,** 1757.

Ley, K., Laudanna, C., Cybulsky, M. I., and Nourshargh, S. (2007). Getting to the site of inflammation: The leukocyte adhesion cascade updated. *Nat. Rev. Immunol.* **7,** 678.

Lim, J. K., Obara, C. J., Rivollier, A., Pletnev, A. G., Kelsall, B. L., and Murphy, P. M. (2011). Chemokine receptor ccr2 is critical for monocyte accumulation and survival in West Nile virus encephalitis. *J. Immunol.* **186,** 471.

MacMicking, J. D., Nathan, C., Hom, G., Chartrain, N., Fletcher, D. S., Trumbauer, M., Stevens, K., Xie, Q. W., Sokol, K., Hutchinson, N., *et al.* (1995). Altered responses to bacterial infection and endotoxic shock in mice lacking inducible nitric oxide synthase. *Cell* **81,** 641.

Mendez-Ferrer, S., Michurina, T. V., Ferraro, F., Mazloom, A. R., Macarthur, B. D., Lira, S. A., Scadden, D. T., Ma'ayan, A., Enikolopov, G. N., and Frenette, P. S. (2010). Mesenchymal and haematopoietic stem cells form a unique bone marrow niche. *Nature* **466,** 829.

Murray, E. G. D., Webb, R. A., and Swann, M. B. R. (1926). A disease of rabbits characterized by a large mononuclear monocytosis, caused by a hitherto undescribed bacillus Bacterium monocytogenes. *J. Pathol. Bacteriol.* **29,** 407.

O'Connell, R. M., Saha, S. K., Vaidya, S. A., Bruhn, K. W., Miranda, G. A., Zarnegar, B., Perry, A. K., Nguyen, B. O., Lane, T. F., Taniguchi, T., Miller, J. F., and Cheng, G. (2004). Type I interferon production enhances susceptibility to Listeria monocytogenes infection. *J. Exp. Med.* **200,** 437.

O'Riordan, M., Yi, C. H., Gonzales, R., Lee, K. D., and Portnoy, D. A. (2002). Innate recognition of bacteria by a macrophage cytosolic surveillance pathway. *Proc. Natl. Acad. Sci. USA* **99,** 13861.

Palframan, R. T., Jung, S., Cheng, G., Weninger, W., Luo, Y., Dorf, M., Littman, D. R., Rollins, B. J., Zweerink, H., Rot, A., and von Andrian, U. H. (2001). Inflammatory chemokine transport and presentation in HEV: A remote control mechanism for monocyte recruitment to lymph nodes in inflamed tissues. *J. Exp. Med.* **194,** 1361.

Pfeffer, K., Matsuyama, T., Kundig, T. M., Wakeham, A., Kishihara, K., Shahinian, A., Wiegmann, K., Ohashi, P. S., Kronke, M., and Mak, T. W. (1993). Mice deficient for the 55 kd tumor necrosis factor receptor are resistant to endotoxic shock, yet succumb to L. monocytogenes infection. *Cell* **73,** 457.

Pirie, J. H. H. (1927). A new disease of veld rodents. "Tiger River Disease". *Publ. S. Afr. Inst. Med. Res.* **3,** 163.

Proudfoot, A. E., Handel, T. M., Johnson, Z., Lau, E. K., LiWang, P., Clark-Lewis, I., Borlat, F., Wells, T. N., and Kosco-Vilbois, M. H. (2003). Glycosaminoglycan binding and oligomerization are essential for the in vivo activity of certain chemokines. *Proc. Natl. Acad. Sci. USA* **100,** 1885.

Rollins, B. J., and Pober, J. S. (1991). Interleukin-4 induces the synthesis and secretion of MCP-1/JE by human endothelial cells. *Am. J. Pathol.* **138,** 1315.

Rosen, H., Gordon, S., and North, R. J. (1989). Exacerbation of murine listeriosis by a monoclonal antibody specific for the type 3 complement receptor of myelomonocytic cells. Absence of monocytes at infective foci allows Listeria to multiply in nonphagocytic cells. *J. Exp. Med.* **170,** 27.

Rothe, J., Lesslauer, W., Lotscher, H., Lang, Y., Koebel, P., Kontgen, F., Althage, A., Zinkernagel, R., Steinmetz, M., and Bluethmann, H. (1993). Mice lacking the tumour necrosis factor receptor 1 are resistant to TNF-mediated toxicity but highly susceptible to infection by Listeria monocytogenes. *Nature* **364,** 798.

Seki, E., Tsutsui, H., Tsuji, N. M., Hayashi, N., Adachi, K., Nakano, H., Futatsugi-Yumikura, S., Takeuchi, O., Hoshino, K., Akira, S., Fujimoto, J., and Nakanishi, K. (2002). Critical roles of myeloid differentiation factor 88-dependent proinflammatory cytokine release in early phase clearance of Listeria monocytogenes in mice. *J. Immunol.* **169,** 3863.

Serbina, N. V., and Pamer, E. G. (2006). Monocyte emigration from bone marrow during bacterial infection requires signals mediated by chemokine receptor CCR2. *Nat. Immunol.* **7,** 311.

Serbina, N. V., Kuziel, W., Flavell, R., Akira, S., Rollins, B., and Pamer, E. G. (2003a). Sequential MyD88-independent and -dependent activation of innate immune responses to intracellular bacterial infection. *Immunity* **19,** 891.

Serbina, N. V., Salazar-Mather, T. P., Biron, C. A., Kuziel, W. A., and Pamer, E. G. (2003b). TNF/iNOS-producing dendritic cells mediate innate immune defense against bacterial infection. *Immunity* **19,** 59.

Serbina, N. V., Jia, T., Hohl, T. M., and Pamer, E. G. (2008). Monocyte-mediated defense against microbial pathogens. *Annu. Rev. Immunol.* **26,** 421.

Serbina, N. V., Hohl, T. M., Cherny, M., and Pamer, E. G. (2009). Selective expansion of the monocytic lineage directed by bacterial infection. *J. Immunol.* **183,** 1900.

Shi, C., Velazquez, P., Hohl, T. M., Leiner, I., Dustin, M. L., and Pamer, E. G. (2010). Monocyte trafficking to hepatic sites of bacterial infection is chemokine independent and directed by focal intercellular adhesion molecule-1 expression. *J. Immunol.* **184,** 6266.

Shi, C., Jia, T., Mendez-Ferrer, S., Hohl, T. M., Serbina, N. V., Lipuma, L., Leiner, I., Li, M. O., Frenette, P. S., and Pamer, E. G. (2011). Bone marrow mesenchymal stem and progenitor cells induce monocyte emigration in response to circulating Toll-like receptor ligands. *Immunity* **34,** 590–601.

Struyf, S., Van Collie, E., Paemen, L., Put, W., Lenaerts, J. P., Proost, P., Opdenakker, G., and Van Damme, J. (1998). Synergistic induction of MCP-1 and -2 by IL-1beta and interferons in fibroblasts and epithelial cells. *J. Leukoc. Biol.* **63,** 364.

Sugiyama, T., Kohara, H., Noda, M., and Nagasawa, T. (2006). Maintenance of the hematopoietic stem cell pool by CXCL12-CXCR4 chemokine signaling in bone marrow stromal cell niches. *Immunity* **25,** 977.

Tripp, C. S., Wolf, S. F., and Unanue, E. R. (1993). Interleukin 12 and tumor necrosis factor alpha are costimulators of interferon gamma production by natural killer cells in severe combined immunodeficiency mice with listeriosis, and interleukin 10 is a physiologic antagonist. *Proc. Natl. Acad. Sci. USA* **90,** 3725.

Tsou, C. L., Peters, W., Si, Y., Slaymaker, S., Aslanian, A. M., Weisberg, S. P., Mack, M., and Charo, I. F. (2007). Critical roles for CCR2 and MCP-3 in monocyte mobilization from bone marrow and recruitment to inflammatory sites. *J. Clin. Invest.* **117,** 902.

Tsuboi, N., Yoshikai, Y., Matsuo, S., Kikuchi, T., Iwami, K., Nagai, Y., Takeuchi, O., Akira, S., and Matsuguchi, T. (2002). Roles of toll-like receptors in C-C chemokine production by renal tubular epithelial cells. *J. Immunol.* **169,** 2026.

CHAPTER 8

Innate Immune Pathways Triggered by *Listeria monocytogenes* and Their Role in the Induction of Cell-Mediated Immunity

Chelsea E. Witte,* Kristina A. Archer,† Chris S. Rae,† John-Demian Sauer,§ Joshua J. Woodward,¶ and Daniel A. Portnoy*,†,‡

Contents

* Graduate Group in Microbiology, University of California, Berkeley, Berkeley, California, USA
† Department of Molecular and Cell Biology, University of California, Berkeley, Berkeley, California, USA
‡ School of Public Health, University of California, Berkeley, Berkeley, California, USA
§ Department of Medical Microbiology and Immunology, University of Wisconsin-Madison, Madison, Wisconsin, USA
¶ Department of Microbiology, University of Washington, Seattle, Washington, USA

Advances in Immunology, Volume 113
ISSN 0065-2776, DOI: 10.1016/B978-0-12-394590-7.00002-6

Abstract

Acquired cell-mediated immunity to *Listeria monocytogenes* is induced by infection with live, replicating bacteria that grow in the host cell cytosol, whereas killed bacteria, or those trapped in a phagosome, fail to induce protective immunity. In this chapter, we focus on how *L. monocytogenes* is sensed by the innate immune system, with the presumption that innate immunity affects the development of acquired immunity. Infection by *L. monocytogenes* induces three innate immune pathways: an MyD88-dependent pathway emanating from a phagosome leading to expression of inflammatory cytokines; a STING/IRF3-dependent pathway emanating from the cytosol leading to the expression of IFN-β and coregulated genes; and very low levels of a Caspase-1-dependent, AIM2-dependent inflammasome pathway resulting in proteolytic activation and secretion of IL-1β and IL-18 and pyroptotic cell death. Using a combination of genetics and biochemistry, we identified the listerial ligand that activates the STING/IRF3 pathway as secreted cyclic diadenosine monophosphate, a newly discovered conserved bacterial signaling molecule. We also identified *L. monocytogenes* mutants that caused robust inflammasome activation due to bacteriolysis in the cytosol, release of DNA, and activation of the AIM2 inflammasome. A strain was constructed that ectopically expressed and secreted a fusion protein containing *Legionella pneumophila* flagellin that robustly activated the Nlrc4-dependent inflammasome and was highly attenuated in mice, also in an Nlrc4-dependent manner. Surprisingly, this strain was a poor inducer of adaptive immunity, suggesting that inflammasome activation is not necessary to induce cell-mediated immunity and may even be detrimental under some conditions. To the best of our knowledge, no single innate immune pathway is necessary to mount a robust acquired immune response to *L. monocytogenes* infection.

1. INTRODUCTION

The year 2012 is the 50th anniversary of the classic work of George Mackaness in which he developed the murine model of listeriosis and showed that resistance and immunity to *L. monocytogenes* infection were mediated by activated macrophages (Mackaness, 1962). Shortly thereafter, he demonstrated that while innate resistance was not specific, acquired immunity was highly specific (Mackaness, 1964), a trait that later was explained by the development of antigen-specific CD8+ T cells (Lane and Unanue, 1972; North, 1973; Pamer, 2004; Unanue, 1997). However, the generation of a protective immune response requires that the bacteria are alive and replicating *in vivo*. (Berche *et al.*, 1987; Lauvau *et al.*, 2001; von Koenig *et al.*, 1982). Indeed, this property has led to the development of live, attenuated *L. monocytogenes*-based vaccine vectors for cancer immunotherapy and infectious disease applications that are very potent at inducing CD8+ T cell responses to *L. monocytogenes* and foreign antigens (Brockstedt and Dubensky, 2008; Gravekamp and Paterson, 2010; see Chapter 6 volume).

What are the features of *L. monocytogenes* infection that lead to such a robust cell-mediated immune response? Clearly, the answer is multifactorial, but in broad terms, is a consequence of the cell biology of infection and the associated innate immune responses. The cell biology of infection has been well documented (Hamon *et al.*, 2006; Portnoy *et al.*, 2002; Tilney and Portnoy, 1989), but the most relevant issue that relates to immunity is that the bacteria escape from a phagosome and grow rapidly in the host cell cytosol. The pore-forming cytolysin listeriolysin O (LLO) is essential for bacterial escape from a phagosome and consequently, pathogenicity (Schnupf and Portnoy, 2007). However, LLO is a double-edged sword; mutants that fail to properly compartmentalize LLO activity to a phagosome kill the infected host cell by necrosis and are rendered avirulent (Schnupf and Portnoy, 2007). Another form of cell death is Caspase-1-dependent cell death termed pyroptosis (Fink and Cookson, 2005). As it will be discussed below, *L. monocytogenes* induces low levels of pyroptosis and mutants engineered to trigger this response are highly attenuated (Sauer *et al.*, 2011a). Thus, to promote its pathogenesis, *L. monocytogenes* must avoid killing its infected host cell. Conversely, one hypothesis that explains the requirement of CD8+ T cells is that the host needs to kill infected cells in order to clear the infection, and indeed, that is a primary function of CD8+ T cells (Harty *et al.*, 2000).

Another essential bacterial determinant of pathogenesis is ActA, a cell surface protein that mediates actin-based motility, thereby promoting bacterial spread intra- and intercellularly (Gouin *et al.*, 2005; Portnoy *et al.*, 2002). ActA-minus mutants, although attenuated, still grow in the host cell cytosol and are potent inducers of immunity. This property has allowed investigators to use ActA-minus mutants to immunize knockout mice that are highly susceptible to wild-type *L. monocytogenes*, including MyD88-, IFN-γ-, and TNF-α-deficient mice (Harty and White, 1999; Way *et al.*, 2003).

Similar to killed bacteria, LLO-minus mutants fail to induce protective immunity (Bahjat *et al.*, 2006; Berche *et al.*, 1987), leading to the hypothesis that cytosolic bacteria are immunogenic due to the secretion of antigens in the cytosol. Indeed, most of the antigens presented in the context of MHC Class I molecules are derived from secreted proteins (Pamer, 2004). In addition, cytosolic bacteria induce a distinct array of cytokines compared to bacteria trapped in a phagosome (Leber *et al.*, 2008; O'Riordan *et al.*, 2002). Therefore, a second hypothesis is that innate immune responses that emanate from detection of cytosolic bacteria may also contribute to the induction of acquired immunity.

It is generally understood that the generation of acquired immunity requires prior induction of innate immunity, and this provides the basis of adjuvant action (Mbow *et al.*, 2010; Schenten and Medzhitov, 2011). In this review, we focus on how the innate immune system recognizes *L. monocytogenes*, with the presumption that innate immunity affects the development of acquired immunity. We will discuss three distinct pathways (Fig. 8.1). The first is an MyD88-dependent pathway that emanates from the cell surface and phagosome, leading to the expression of inflammatory and suppressive/regulatory cytokines such as TNF-α, IL-12, and IL-10 (Gilchrist *et al.*, 2006; Kawai and Akira, 2010; Kobayashi *et al.*, 2005). The second pathway emanates from the cytosol and is dependent on STING and IRF3, leading to the robust expression of IFN-β and coregulated genes (Barber, 2011). The third pathway is Caspase-1-dependent inflammasome activation that results in the proteolytic activation and secretion of IL-1β and IL-18 and eventually to pyroptotic cell death (Martinon *et al.*, 2009). We will provide evidence that *L. monocytogenes* induces pyroptosis, however, infrequently (Sauer *et al.*, 2010). In fact, *L. monocytogenes* strains

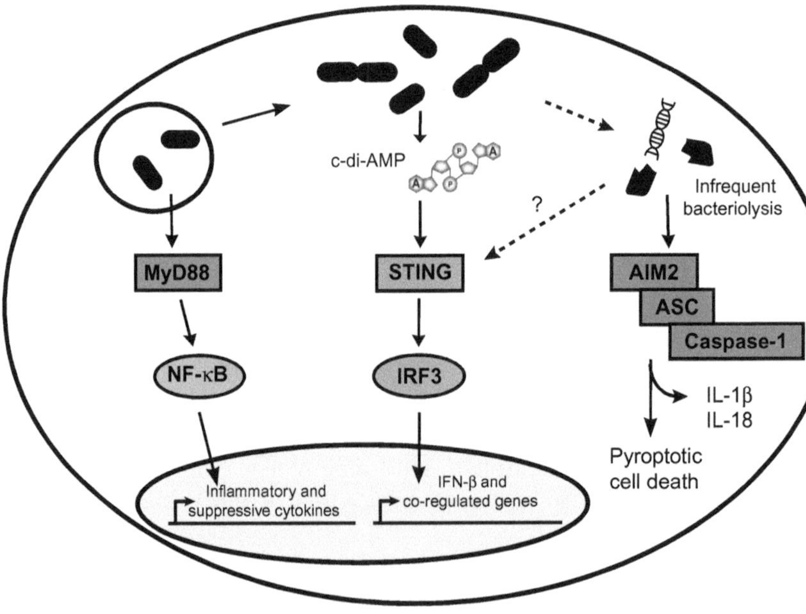

FIGURE 8.1 Innate immune pathways triggered by *L. monocytogenes*. During infection of macrophages, *L. monocytogenes* is detected by three distinct innate immune pathways: one that is dependent on MyD88, one that is dependent on STING/IRF3, and an AIM-2-mediated inflammasome pathway. Each pathway results in a distinct host response to infection. Dashed lines represent infrequent events. (See Color Insert.)

engineered to robustly activate the inflammasome are avirulent and induce diminished protective immunity (Sauer *et al.*, 2011a).

2. INNATE IMMUNE RESPONSES TO *L. MONOCYTOGENES*

It is generally appreciated that host cells detect microorganisms by stimulation of a family of receptors collectively referred to as the Toll-like receptors (TLRs) (Beutler *et al.*, 2006; Kawai and Akira, 2010). TLR activation is triggered by a relatively small number of conserved microbial molecules that in many cases are essential to the *in vivo* survival of the microorganism. TLRs are divided into those present on the surface of host cells and those that localize to a vacuolar compartment (Barbalat *et al.*, 2011). Examples of the former are TLRs 2, 4, and 5, which are triggered by a variety of molecules, most notably, lipopeptides, LPS, and flagellin, respectively. The TLRs that signal from endosomal compartments include TLRs 3, 7, and 9, each of which is stimulated by nucleic acids (Barbalat *et al.*, 2011). Engagement of TLRs by their ligand(s) triggers a signal transduction cascade that mediates expression of molecules associated with inflammation. Two important adaptor proteins contribute to TLR-dependent signaling: MyD88 is required for signaling downstream of the majority of TLRs, while Trif acts downstream of TLR3 leading to a distinct expression profile that includes IFN-β and coregulated genes. TLR4 is the only known receptor that can use either adaptor, although only Trif-dependent signaling leads to a distinct transcriptional response that includes the expression of IFN-β. While MyD88 contributes to surface and vacuolar signaling, there is evidence that Trif-dependent signaling emanates from an endosomal compartment (Kagan *et al.*, 2008).

Transcriptional profiling of macrophages infected with *L. monocytogenes* reveals a complex pattern of host gene expression that involves hundreds of genes (Leber *et al.*, 2008; McCaffrey *et al.*, 2004) (Fig. 8.2). Multiple innate immune pathways often overlap in their response, but this can often be sorted out by using both bacterial and host mutants, so-called genetics squared (Persson and Vance, 2007). For example, MyD88-deficient macrophages have no significant response to LLO-minus bacteria suggesting that the innate immune response to mutants that are trapped in a phagosome is entirely mediated by MyD88 (Fig. 8.2). MyD88-dependent responses are clearly important for host resistance, as MyD88-deficient mice are extremely sensitive to *L. monocytogenes* infection, implying that TLR-dependent recognition plays an important role in host defense (Edelson and Unanue, 2002; Way *et al.*, 2003). So, what are the bacterial ligands that trigger a MyD88-dependent response and which TLRs are involved? On the host side, TLR2 is a good candidate, as it can be stimulated by a number of potential *L. monocytogenes* ligands including

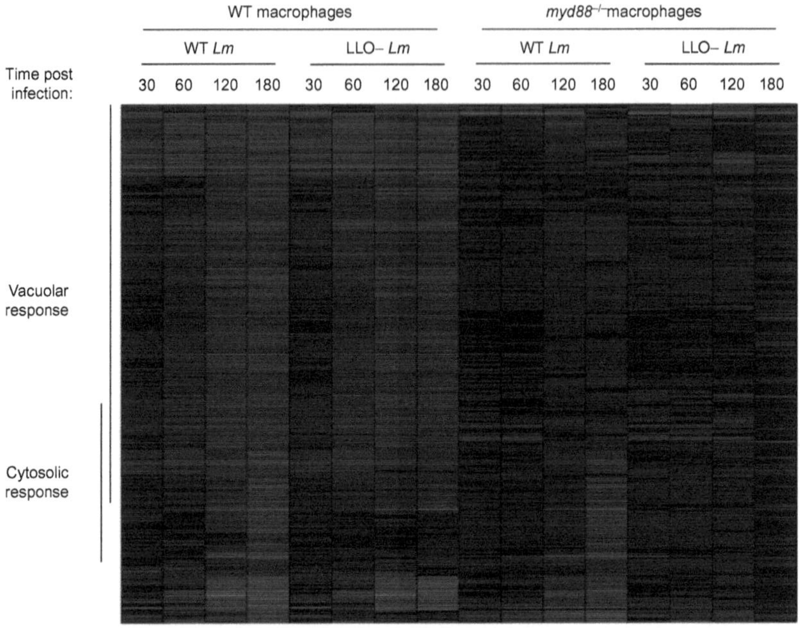

FIGURE 8.2 Macrophages have distinct transcriptional responses to vacuolar and cytosolic *L. monocytogenes* infection. Adapted from Leber *et al.* (2008). Cluster analysis of the microarrary determination of all mouse macrophage genes with at least fourfold change in abundance during infection of wild-type and MyD88-deficient macrophages with either wild-type or LLO-minus *L. monocytogenes*, at the indicated times postinfection (minutes). Red indicates an increase in RNA abundance relative to uninfected macrophages, and green indicates a decrease. Genes identified by significant analysis of microarrays (SAM) and at least fourfold induced in wild-type macrophages by LLO-minus *L. monocytogenes* are indicated as targets of the "vacuolar response." Genes identified by SAM and at least fourfold induced in MyD88-deficient macrophages by wild-type *L. monocytogenes* are indicated as targets of the "cytosolic response" (Leber *et al.*, 2008). (See Color Insert.)

lipoteichoic acid, lipoproteins, and potentially peptidoglycan (Dziarski and Gupta, 2010; Travassos *et al.*, 2004). However, *in vivo*, TLR2-deficient mice are either fully resistant or exhibit only mild susceptibility upon infection, indicating that TLR2 is not the only MyD88-dependent TLR triggered by *L. monocytogenes* (Edelson and Unanue, 2002; Janot *et al.*, 2008; Torres *et al.*, 2004). *L. monocytogenes* flagellin stimulates TLR5 (Hayashi *et al.*, 2001) and may play a role under some conditions, but TLR5 is not expressed in murine macrophages (Uematsu *et al.*, 2006), and therefore plays no apparent role in our analysis. TLR4 is unlikely to contribute to the recognition of *L. monocytogenes*, as its major ligand, LPS, is not present in Gram-positive bacteria, including *L. monocytogenes*.

Signaling from all of the vacuolar TLRs, but not the surface TLRs, requires a transmembrane protein named Unc93b (Tabeta *et al.*, 2006) that traffics from the endoplasmic reticulum to TLR-containing endosomal compartments (Barbalat *et al.*, 2011). Macrophages from Unc93b-deficient mice show reduced expression of IL-12 and TNF-α upon infection with LLO-minus bacteria (Tabeta *et al.*, 2006), suggesting that *L. monocytogenes* nucleic acids may contribute to the MyD88-dependent response. In addition, *L. monocytogenes* mutants that are sensitive to lysozyme are degraded in a phagosome and stimulate higher levels of MyD88-dependent cytokines than wild-type bacteria (Boneca *et al.*, 2007; Rae *et al.*, 2011). Taken together, these data suggest that multiple *L. monocytogenes* ligands recognized at both the host cell surface and within a vacuole contribute to the MyD88-dependent response to *L. monocytogenes*.

As discussed in detail in later sections, it is clear that wild-type *L. monocytogenes* trigger a pathway of host gene expression that is referred to as the cytosolic surveillance pathway (CSP) (O'Riordan *et al.*, 2002). Expression of the CSP requires STING and IRF3, so we will refer to this as a STING/IRF3-dependent response (Barber, 2011; Jin *et al.*, 2011; Sauer *et al.*, 2011b). There are nearly two-dozen primary genes that are induced by this pathway, but the most highly upregulated IRF3-dependent gene is IFN-β (Leber *et al.*, 2008). Thus, measuring IFN-β by using either an IFN-dependent luciferase reporter (L929-ISRE cells) or a qRT-PCR serves as a convenient readout for this response. Importantly, the CSP is induced by a variety of other intracellular pathogens, including *Mycobacterium tuberculosis, Legionella pneumophila,* and *Francisella tularensis* (Vance *et al.*, 2009).

3. IDENTIFICATION OF BACTERIAL MUTANTS THAT INDUCE DIMINISHED OR ENHANCED INDUCTION OF THE CYTOSOLIC SURVEILLANCE PATHWAY AND/OR INFLAMMASOME ACTIVATION

3.1. A genetic screen to identify bacterial mutants

Although the host pathways of cytosolic bacterial recognition are becoming better defined, until recently, none of the listerial ligands responsible for this response had been identified. DNA transfected into macrophages recapitulated the response leading to the expression of IFN-β, but there was no evidence that this represented the endogenous ligand (Leber *et al.*, 2008; Stetson and Medzhitov, 2006). To gain an appreciation of bacterial ligands that stimulate the CSP, our laboratory developed a comprehensive forward genetic screen to identify bacterial mutants that induced, enhanced, or diminished levels of IFN-β expression and/or host cell death (Fig. 8.3).

Prior to the screen, libraries of *L. monocytogenes* transposon mutants were constructed using either a *Tn917* derivative (Camilli *et al.*, 1990) or more recently a *Himar1 mariner* transposon (Zemansky *et al.*, 2009). The design of the new *Himar1* transposon minimizes polar effects, and its

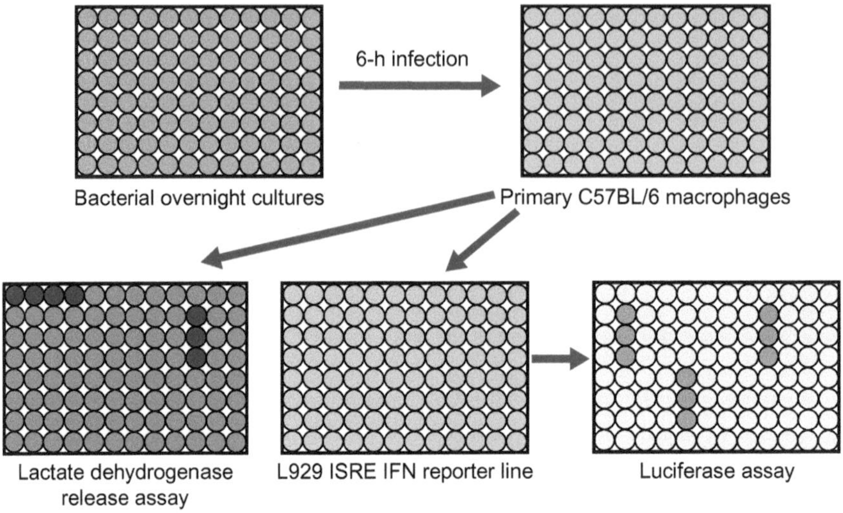

FIGURE 8.3 Schematic of genetic screen. *L. monocytogenes* transposon insertion mutants were grown overnight and used to infect primary bone marrow-derived macrophages. Following 6 h of infection, supernatants from the infected cells were analyzed for IFN-β stimulation by L929-ISRE reporter cells, which produce luciferase in response to IFN-β, as well as for host cell death as measured by lactate dehydrogenase release. (See Color Insert.)

low-site specificity eliminates insertional ''hot spots,'' providing full genomic coverage. Isolated mutants were grown to stationary phase overnight at 30°C and used to infect primary, bone marrow-derived murine macrophages. Following 6 hours of infection, supernatants from the infected macrophages were harvested and used to assess each mutant's ability to induce (i) the STING/IRF3-dependent pathway as measured by IFN-β production and (ii) lactate dehydrogenase (LDH) release, which is a consequence of inflammasome activation and pyroptotic cell death. *In vitro* secondary screening for motility and hemolysis eliminated mutations that affected infectivity or phagosomal escape of the bacteria. Mutants identified in the screen can be classified into three groups: those that affected IFN-β production, those that induced altered levels of cell death, or those that affected both cytosolic signaling pathways (Table 8.1). Examination of Table 8.1 reveals a number of phenotypes that although, reproducible, are currently unexplainable.

3.2. Identification of ligands that induce the CSP

Three of the mutants isolated from the screen-harbored transposon insertions in genes predicted to encode negative transcriptional regulators of bacterial multidrug resistance transporters (MDRs) (Crimmins *et al.*, 2008).

TABLE 8.1 *L. monocytogenes* transposon mutants identified in forward genetic screens for stimulation of IFN-β and host cell death

L. monocytogenes gene harboring transposon insertion	Strain number	Description	Fold IFN-β induction[a]	Fold host cell death[b]	Relative bacteriolysis[c]	Reference
Mutants that affected IFN-β production						
lmo0052	DP-L5896	Cyclic di-AMP phosphodiesterase	5.0	NS	0.5	
lmo0165	DP-L5897	Predicted *O*-methyltransferase	0.4	NS	1.0	
lmo0559	DP-L5507	Pgl, 6-phosphoglu conolactonase	3.0	NS	ND	Crimmins *et al.* (2009)
lmo0583	DP-L5898	Similar to preprotein translocase SecA subunit	1.6	NS	0.5	
lmo0597	DP-L5899	Similar to transcriptional regulator, CRF/FNR family	2.3	NS	1.2	
lmo0781	DP-L5900	Similar to mannose-specific phosphotransferase component IID	2.4	NS	1.4	
lmo0847	DP-L5901	Similar to glutamine ABC transporter	0.4	NS	0.7	
lmo1348	DP-L5902	GcvT, glycine cleavage system aminomethyltransferase	0.4	NS	10.2	
lmo1408	DP-L5396	LadR, negative regulator of MDR transporter, MdrL	3.0	NS	ND	Crimmins *et al.* (2008)

(*continued*)

TABLE 8.1 (*continued*)

L. monocytogenes gene harboring transposon insertion	Strain number	Description	Fold IFN-β induction[a]	Fold host cell death[b]	Relative bacteriolysis[c]	Reference
Δ lmo1617	DP-L5444	MdrM, MDR transporter	0.3	NS	ND	Crimmins *et al.* (2008)
lmo1745	DP-L5398	VirR, putative two-component system response regulator	3.0	NS	ND	
lmo2114	DP-L5903	Similar to ABC transporter (ATP-binding protein)	1.7	NS	1.1	
lmo2477	DP-L5904	GalE, UDP-glucose 4-epimerase	1.8	NS	1.9	
lmo2589	DP-L5397	TetR, negative regulator of MDR transporter, MdrT	20.0	NS	ND	Crimmins *et al.* (2008)
lmo2691	DP-L5905	Autolysin, *N*-acetyl muramidase	1.8	NS	1.9	
lmo2783	DP-L5906	Similar to cellobiose phosphotransferase system, component IIC	1.5	NS	4.6	
Mutants that affected host cell death						
lmo0540	DP-L5907	Similar to penicillin-binding protein	NS	1.8	1.8	
lmo0687	DP-L5908	Hypothetical protein	NS	1.8	2.8	
lmo0692	DP-L5909	CheA, two-component sensor histidine kinase, involved in chemotaxis	NS	0.5	0.6	

TABLE 8.1 *(continued)*

L. monocytogenes gene harboring transposon insertion	Strain number	Description	Fold IFN-β induction[a]	Fold host cell death[b]	Relative bacteriolysis[c]	Reference
lmo0785	DP-L5910	Similar to transcriptional regulator, NifA/NtrC family	NS	1.6	0.2	
lmo0893	DP-L5911	RsbV, anti-anti-sigma factor	NS	0.5	1.5	
lmo2474	DP-L5912	Hypothetical protein	NS	4.4	7.2	
lmo2638	DP-L5913	Similar to NADH dehydrogenase	NS	2.5	0.7	
lmo2639	DP-L5914	Hypothetical protein	NS	1.9	0.7	
Mutants that affected both IFN-β and host cell death						
lmo0707	DP-L5915	FliD, flagellar capping protein	1.9	2.3	2.9	
lmo1746	DP-L5916	Similar to ABC transporter, permease	1.5	1.9	1.4	
lmo2045	DP-L5917	Hypothetical protein	2.0	2.5	0.7	
lmo2167	DP-L5918	Hypothetical protein	1.5	0.4	0.3	
lmo2473	DP-L5919	Hypothetical protein, similar to *B. subtilis* YvcK	2.7	4.0	19.7	Sauer *et al*. (2010)
lmo2503	DP-L5920	Similar to cardiolipin synthase	1.9	2.0	0.8	
lmo2554	DP-L5921	Similar to galactosyltransferase	1.3	2.0	3.4	

Values are represented as fold induction compared to infection with wild-type *L. monocytogenes*.
ND, no data. NS, not significantly different compared to wild-type *L. monocytogenes*.
[a] IFN-β induction was quantified either by qRT-PCR on RNA isolated from infected macrophages or by bioassay on supernatants from infected macrophages.
[b] Host cell death was measured by lactate dehydrogenase release into the supernatant of infected macrophages.
[c] Relative bacteriolysis was measured by luminescence as indirect readout of host expression of the reporter plasmid, pBH573, as previously described (Sauer *et al*., 2010).

The insertions in *ladR* (*lmo1408*) and *tetR* (*lmo2589*, later renamed *brtA* (Quillin *et al.*, 2011)) led to transcriptional upregulation of their cognate MDR transporters, *mdrL* (*lmo1409*) and *mdrT* (*lmo2588*), respectively, and resulted in hyperstimulation of IFN-β production. The transposon insertion in *marR* (*lmo1618*), the negative regulator of *mdrM* (*lmo1617*), was located near the 3′ end of the *marR* gene and disrupted expression of *mdrM* directly downstream. Infection with this mutant resulted in decreased expression of IFN-β compared to infection with wild-type *L. monocytogenes* indicating that MDR expression is critical for the IFN-β response. Based on these results, we hypothesized that upregulation of MDRs facilitated the transport of a bacterial ligand into the host cytosol that resulted in host IFN-β production. In contrast, downregulation of MDRs, as in the case of the transposon insertion in *marR* or a deletion of *mdrM*, prevented transport of the ligand and hence induced less IFN-β compared to wild-type *L. monocytogenes*. Nevertheless, even the MdrM-minus mutants induced detectable levels of IFN-β indicating that there is either an MdrM-independent mechanism to secrete cyclic diadenosine monophosphate (c-di-AMP) or another STING-dependent ligand, likely DNA.

All of the MDRs identified in the screen are members of the major facilitator superfamily (MFS) of MDRs (Lewinson *et al.*, 2006). Based on the known properties of MFS family members, we predicted that the ligand would be less than 2 kDa. Further, with the exception of LPS, all known ligands that induce the expression of IFN-β are nucleic acids (Barbalat *et al.*, 2011); therefore, we hypothesized that the ligand would be a small nucleic acid. We used bacterial mutants overexpressing MDRs and HPLC fractionation of culture supernatants to identify an active fraction that stimulated the CSP upon introduction into cells by digitonin permeabilization. This active fraction was analyzed by mass spectrometry and shown to contain c-di-AMP (Woodward *et al.*, 2010). Commercially available synthetic c-di-AMP similarly activated the response. Interestingly, a related bacterial signaling molecule, c-di-GMP, also activates the CSP (McWhirter *et al.*, 2009). Induction of IFN-β by either cyclic di-nucleotide is STING-dependent *in vitro* and *in vivo* (Jin *et al.*, 2011; Sauer *et al.*, 2011b). In addition, it was recently demonstrated that STING functions as the host receptor for cyclic dinucleotides (Burdette *et al.*, 2011).

Additionally, we isolated a mutant harboring a transposon insertion in *lmo0052*, which was initially predicted to encode a hypothetical protein (C. E. Witte, J. D. Sauer, D. A. Portnoy, unpublished data). This mutant induced nearly fivefold more IFN-β compared to infection with wild-type *L. monocytogenes*. Based on homology to the *Bacillus subtilis* protein YybT (Rao *et al.*, 2010) and biochemical characterization, we determined that *lmo0052* encodes a c-di-AMP phosphodiesterase (Pde) (C. E. Witte, J. D. Sauer, D. A. Portnoy, unpublished observations). Transposon inactivation of *lmo0052* is predicted to prevent degradation of c-di-AMP, thereby leading to the accumulation of high levels of c-di-AMP and therefore higher levels of IFN-β induction.

C-di-AMP was only recently discovered where it was found in the crystal structure of a *B. subtilis* sporulation protein called DisA (Witte *et al.*, 2008). DisA has two domains: a DNA-binding domain and a domain with diadenylate cyclase (DAC) activity. *L. monocytogenes lmo2120* has homology to the DAC domain, and its overexpression leads to enhanced levels of IFN-β in infected cells (Woodward *et al.*, 2010). Homologous DAC domains are found in many Gram-positive bacteria including the firmicutes and *M. tuberculosis*, in some Gram-negative bacteria including *Chlamydia* and Spirochetes, and in Archaea (Romling, 2008). The predicted DAC-encoding genes are thought to be essential in *Mycoplasma, Staphylococci,* and *Streptococci* (Forsyth *et al.*, 2002; French *et al.*, 2008; Glass *et al.*, 2006; Song *et al.*, 2005). Thus, c-di-AMP is a conserved and often essential small bacterial signaling molecule that is detected by the host innate immune system. It is not known if c-di-AMP produced by any other bacteria is secreted or detected by the STING/IRF3 innate immune pathway *in vivo.*

3.3. Identification of ligands that induce inflammasome-mediated pyroptotic host cell death

There have been many recent reports that *L. monocytogenes* activates the inflammasome via three different cytosolic sensors: Nlrp3, Nlrc4, and/or AIM2 (Franchi and Nunez, 2010; Franchi *et al.*, 2007; Kim *et al.*, 2010; Mariathasan *et al.*, 2006; Sauer *et al.*, 2010; Warren *et al.*, 2008, 2010; Wu *et al.*, 2010). However, in our hands, the amount of inflammasome-mediated pyroptosis by wild-type *L. monocytogenes* is less than 5% of the infected cells in nonstimulated bone marrow-derived macrophages and approximately 15% in TLR2-prestimulated cells. The release of IL-1β is equally low (Sauer *et al.*, 2010). The increase observed in TLR2-stimulated cells is likely due to induction of inflammasome components and increased phagocytosis. The discrepancy in the literature is probably due to differences in protocols such as multiplicities of infection and the duration of experiments. We feel strongly that, on a cell basis, inflammasome activation in response to *L. monocytogenes* is quite low even during infections with greater than 25 bacteria per cell (Sauer *et al.*, 2010).

To examine *L. monocytogenes* determinants that affect host cell death, we screened the *Himar1* transposon library for mutants that triggered enhanced or diminished host cell death as measured by LDH release (Sauer *et al.*, 2010). Mutants with insertions in *lmo2473* induced fivefold higher cell death, fivefold higher IL-1β secretion, and almost three times the amount of IFN-β compared to wild-type *L. monocytogenes*. This mutant also showed a growth defect in macrophages independent of inflammasome activation that was due to bacteriolysis in the host cell cytosol.

Indeed, other mutants that caused host cell death also showed evidence for increased bacteriolysis in the host cell cytosol. Intracellular bacteriolysis could result in the release of many bacterial ligands, including DNA. Indeed, inflammasome activation induced by *L. monocytogenes* mutants lacking *lmo2473* was abrogated in AIM2-deficient cells, while a control strain engineered to activate the Nlrc4-dependent inflammasome was unaffected in AIM2-deficient cells (J. D. Sauer, and D. A. Portnoy, unpublished data). AIM2 is a cytosolic receptor that mediates DNA-dependent inflammasome activation (Franchi and Nunez, 2010). The low amount of inflammasome activation caused by wild-type *L. monocytogenes* was also largely AIM2 dependent, partially Nlrc4 dependent, and Nlrp3 independent (Sauer *et al.*, 2010). If one assumes that a single lysed bacterium can trigger AIM2-dependent pyroptosis, we estimate that during wild-type infection, less than 1% of the bacteria lyse during intracytosolic growth *in vitro*. However, this amount of lysis results in approximately 5–10% of infected cells undergoing inflammasome activation and pyroptosis (Sauer *et al.*, 2010).

Several mutants identified in the screen had defects in the assembly of bacterial flagella. For example, *lmo0707* encodes a flagellar capping protein (FliD) and mutants defective for FliD are predicted to secrete flagellin. Similarly, *L. monocytogenes* mutants in *flgK*, a flagellar hook-associated component, also secrete flagellin and induced cell death, and in both cases, cell death was Nlrc4 dependent (Warren *et al.*, 2008). Although mutants that misregulate flagella assembly and inappropriately secrete monomers hyperstimulate the Nlrc4 inflammasome, we find a negligible role for Nlrc4-mediated cell death during wild-type infection, which is consistent with the observation that under most conditions, *L. monocytogenes* downregulates flagellar expression at 37 °C (Shen and Higgins, 2006).

Our premise is that *L. monocytogenes* avoids robust inflammasome activation in order to establish infection. We tested this hypothesis by forcing *L. monocytogenes* to activate the inflammasome and observe the effect of inflammasome stimulation on pathogenesis. To accomplish this, a *L. monocytogenes* strain was engineered to secrete a fusion of the N-terminus of the ActA protein linked to the *L. pneumophila* flagellin (Lp-Fla) protein, a potent and well-characterized inducer of the Nlrc4/NAIP5 inflammasome (Sauer *et al.*, 2011a). Unlike wild-type bacteria, the Lp-Fla-expressing strain induced high levels of cell death and IL-1β secretion. Importantly, this strain behaved like wild type in Nlrc4- and Caspase-1-deficient macrophages. The Lp-Fla-expressing strain was highly attenuated in mice, but its pathogenicity was restored in Nlrc4- and Caspase-1-deficient mice. Similar data were also reported by Warren *et al.* (2010) using a very similar inflammasome-activating system. These data suggest that inflammasome activation, at least Nlrc4-mediated, is detrimental to *L. monocytogenes* pathogenesis. Further, these data reinforce the concept that *L. monocytogenes* and perhaps many other intracellular pathogens, such as *Salmonella typhimurium* (Miao *et al.*, 2010), cannot afford to kill their infected host cell.

4. RELATIONSHIP BETWEEN INNATE AND ACQUIRED IMMUNITY

4.1. Role of MyD88 signaling

Although it has been established that cytosolic entry by *L. monocytogenes* is required for the generation of adaptive immunity (Bahjat *et al.*, 2006; Berche *et al.*, 1987; Lauvau *et al.*, 2001; Orgun and Way, 2008), the innate immune components necessary for a robust CD8+ T cell-mediated memory response have yet to be determined. MyD88-deficient mice are highly susceptible to infection with wild-type bacteria, but not with highly attenuated ActA-minus mutants (Way *et al.*, 2003). MyD88-deficient mice immunized with ActA-minus mutants acquired wild-type levels of immunity upon lethal challenge with wild-type bacteria (Way *et al.*, 2003), indicating that TLR activation by phagosomal bacteria is not essential for the induction of protective immunity to *L. monocytogenes*. On the contrary, MyD88-dependent responses may suppress immunity. To evaluate this possibility, Bahjat *et al.* (2009) tested, which was dominant, an ActA-minus strain that induced robust immunity or a LLO-minus strain that failed to induce immunity. Mice were immunized with a relatively high dose of the ActA-minus strain (10^6 CFUs) in the presence of increasing doses of the LLO-minus strain ranging from 10^6 to 10^8 CFUs. Surprisingly, the LLO-minus strain dramatically decreased the levels of immunity induced by the ActA-minus strain. However, in MyD88-deficient mice, there was virtually no suppression. Further, there was little suppression if a blocking antibody to the IL-10 receptor was injected prior to immunization, suggesting that IL-10 secretion in response to LLO-minus immunization could be responsible for inhibiting acquired immunity. Although MyD88 clearly promotes immunity under some experimental conditions (Seubert *et al.*, 2011), our data support the notion that MyD88-dependent signaling is not necessary for the induction of immunity to *L. monocytogenes* but instead may be suppressive.

4.2. Role of the STING/IRF3 pathway

As MyD88-dependent responses are not required for the induction of anti-*L. monocytogenes* immunity (Way *et al.*, 2003), it is reasonable to hypothesize that the CSP plays a role in the generation of protective immunity. Further, c-di-AMP may represent an endogenous listerial ligand acting as an adjuvant. Indeed, there is evidence that cyclic dinucleotides have strong immunostimulatory properties (Chen *et al.*, 2010; Karaolis *et al.*, 2007). C-di-AMP, c-di-GMP, and cyclic di-inosine monophosphate induce dendritic cells to upregulate the surface expression of costimulatory molecules *in vitro* (Libanova *et al.*, 2010; Madhun *et al.*, 2011). In addition, mice immunized with a protein antigen in the presence of c-di-GMP or c-di-AMP produce higher levels of antigen-specific antibodies than mice immunized with protein alone. Splenocytes isolated from these immunized mice proliferate and secrete inflammatory cytokines when peptide stimulated *ex vivo* (Ebensen *et al.*, 2007; Karaolis *et al.*, 2007; McWhirter *et al.*, 2009). C-di-GMP has also been shown to protect against primary bacterial infection (Karaolis *et al.*, 2007; Ogunniyi *et al.*, 2008). Mice immunized with either the avirulent *Staphylococcus aureus* or the protein ClfA in the presence of c-di-GMP have reduced bacterial loads and higher survival rates when challenged with virulent *S. aureus* compared to mice immunized with c-di-GMP alone (Hu *et al.*, 2009). Thus, it is clear that cyclic dinucleotides have adjuvant properties both *in vitro* and *in vivo*, yet whether these heightened innate immune responses contribute to the induction of CD8+ T cell responses and adaptive immunity to *L. monocytogenes* remains unknown.

4.3. Role of inflammasome activation

Little is known about the relationship between inflammasome activation and induction of acquired immunity. However, there is accumulating evidence that some adjuvants act by stimulating the inflammasome leading to enhanced antibody production (Eisenbarth and Flavell, 2009; Eisenbarth *et al.*, 2008; Korn *et al.*, 2009; Kumar *et al.*, 2009; Meng *et al.*, 2009; Watanabe *et al.*, 2008). In addition, inflammasome activation plays an important role in immunity to influenza virus (Allen *et al.*, 2009; Ichinohe *et al.*, 2009). As *L. monocytogenes* induces relatively low levels of inflammasome activation, it is reasonable to suspect that inflammasome activation is not necessary for the induction of protective immunity. Supporting this hypothesis, Caspase-1-deficient mice are immunized as well as wild-type mice by both sub-lethal doses of wild-type *L. monocytogenes* and ActA-minus mutants (Sauer *et al.*, 2011a).

To directly evaluate the role of inflammasome activation, we used the strain described above that secretes a fusion of ActA and Lp-Fla (Sauer *et al.*, 2011a). Surprisingly, this strain was a poor inducer of adaptive immunity, both at the level of antigen-specific T cell development and induction of long-lived protective immunity. Therefore, we conclude that inflammasome activation, at least in the case of the Nlrc4 inflammasome, is not necessary to induce immunity and may even be detrimental. One possibility is that inflammasome-activating strains kill infected dendritic cells, thereby affecting T cell priming.

5. CONCLUSIONS AND FUTURE PROSPECTS

Returning to a modified version of the question posed at the beginning of this review: what, if any, innate immune pathway contributes to the capacity of *L. monocytogenes* to induce such a robust cell-mediated immune response? Our original hypothesis was that one of the three innate immune pathways depicted in Fig. 8.1 would be critical for the induction of protective immunity. However, neither MyD88, Caspase-1, nor the type I IFN receptor is necessary for the development of acquired immunity to *L. monocytogenes* (Sauer *et al.*, 2011a; Way *et al.*, 2003). The role of STING or c-di-AMP has not been evaluated, but preliminary data from our lab indicates that STING-deficient mice also develop immunity to *L. monocytogenes*. Thus, removal of any one of the three innate pathways shown in Fig. 8.1 has no clear affect on the generation of immunity. Although there are many innate immune pathways necessary for resistance to primary infection, we are currently not aware of a mouse deficient in a single innate immune pathway that is unable to mount robust immunity to *L. monocytogenes*. The simplest explanation is that of redundancy. Perhaps any source of inflammation that occurs in the context of cytosolic antigen delivery by *L. monocytogenes* triggers protective T cell development, while hyperinduction of any single pathway leads to a diminished response. Indeed, it has been suggested that, under some experimental conditions, inflammation plays a negative role in priming a CD8+ T cell memory response (Harty and Badovinac, 2008). In the future, studies using a combination of bacterial and host mutants altered in one or more innate immune pathway will shed light on the precise requirements for the induction of immunity.

ACKNOWLEDGMENTS

This work was supported by the Ruth L. Kirschstein National Research Service Award (5F32AI084333 to K. A. A.), American Cancer Society (PF-07-066-01-LIB to J. D. S), and National Institute of Health (F32 A184372 to J. J. W.; 1RO1 AI27655 and 1PO1 AI63302 to D. A. P).

D. A. P. has a consulting relationship with and a financial interest in Aduro BioTech, Berkeley, CA.

REFERENCES

Allen, I. C., Scull, M. A., Moore, C. B., Holl, E. K., McElvania-TeKippe, E., Taxman, D. J., Guthrie, E. H., Pickles, R. J., and Ting, J. P. (2009). The NLRP3 inflammasome mediates in vivo innate immunity to influenza A virus through recognition of viral RNA. *Immunity* **30**, 556.

Bahjat, K. S., Liu, W., Lemmens, E. E., Schoenberger, S. P., Portnoy, D. A., Dubensky, T. W., Jr., and Brockstedt, D. G. (2006). Cytosolic entry controls CD8+ T-cell potency during bacterial infection. *Infect. Immun.* **74,** 6387.

Bahjat, K. S., Meyer-Morse, N., Lemmens, E. E., Shugart, J. A., Dubensky, T. W., Brockstedt, D. G., and Portnoy, D. A. (2009). Suppression of cell-mediated immunity following recognition of phagosome-confined bacteria. *PLoS Pathog.* **5,** e1000568.

Barbalat, R., Ewald, S. E., Mouchess, M. L., and Barton, G. M. (2011). Nucleic acid recognition by the innate immune system. *Annu. Rev. Immunol.* **29,** 185.

Barber, G. N. (2011). Innate immune DNA sensing pathways: STING, AIMII and the regulation of interferon production and inflammatory responses. *Curr. Opin. Immunol.* **23,** 10.

Berche, P., Gaillard, J., and Sansonetti, P. J. (1987). Intracellular growth of Listeria monocytogenes as a prerequisit for in vivo induction of T cell-mediated immunity. *J. Immunol.* **138,** 2266.

Beutler, B., Jiang, Z., Georgel, P., Crozat, K., Croker, B., Rutschmann, S., Du, X., and Hoebe, K. (2006). Genetic analysis of host resistance: Toll-like receptor signaling and immunity at large. *Annu. Rev. Immunol.* **24,** 353.

Boneca, I. G., Dussurget, O., Cabanes, D., Nahori, M. A., Sousa, S., Lecuit, M., Psylinakis, E., Bouriotis, V., Hugot, J. P., Giovannini, M., Coyle, A., Bertin, J., *et al.* (2007). A critical role for peptidoglycan N-deacetylation in Listeria evasion from the host innate immune system. *Proc. Natl. Acad. Sci. USA* **104,** 997.

Brockstedt, D. G., and Dubensky, T. W. (2008). Promises and challenges for the development of Listeria monocytogenes-based immunotherapies. *Expert Rev. Vaccines* **7,** 1069.

Burdette, D. L., Monroe, K. M., Sotelo-Troha, K., Iwig, J. S., Eckert, B., Hyodo, M., Hayakawa, Y., and Vance, R. E. (2011). STING is a direct innate immune sensor of cyclic di-GMP. *Nature* **478,** 515–518.

Camilli, A., Portnoy, A., and Youngman, P. (1990). Insertional mutagenesis of Listeria monocytogenes with a novel Tn917 derivative that allows direct cloning of DNA flanking transposon insertions. *J. Bacteriol.* **172,** 3738.

Chen, W., Kuolee, R., and Yan, H. (2010). The potential of 3′,5′-cyclic diguanylic acid (c-di-GMP) as an effective vaccine adjuvant. *Vaccine* **28,** 3080.

Crimmins, G. T., Herskovits, A. A., Rehder, K., Sivick, K. E., Lauer, P., Dubensky, T. W., Jr., and Portnoy, D. A. (2008). Listeria monocytogenes multidrug resistance transporters activate a cytosolic surveillance pathway of innate immunity. *Proc. Natl. Acad. Sci. USA* **105,** 10191.

Crimmins, G. T., Schelle, M. W., Herskovits, A. A., Ni, P. P., Meyer-Morse, N., Ivarone, A. T., and Portnoy, D. A. (2009). *Listeria monocytogenes* 6-phosphogluconolactonase (*pgl*) mutants induce increased activation of a host cytosolic surveillance pathway. *Infect. Immun.* **77,** 3014.

Dziarski, R., and Gupta, D. (2010). Review: Mammalian peptidoglyan recognition proteins (PGRPs) in innate immunity. *Innate Immun.* **16,** 168.

Ebensen, T., Schulze, K., Riese, P., Morr, M., and Guzman, C. A. (2007). The bacterial second messenger cdiGMP exhibits promising activity as a mucosal adjuvant. *Clin. Vaccine Immunol.* **14,** 952.

Edelson, B. T., and Unanue, E. R. (2002). MyD88-dependent but Toll-like receptor 2-independent innate immunity to Listeria: no role for either in macrophage listericidal activity. *J. Immunol.* **169,** 3869.

Eisenbarth, S. C., and Flavell, R. A. (2009). Innate instruction of adaptive immunity revisited: the inflammasome. *EMBO Mol. Med.* **1,** 92.

Eisenbarth, S. C., Colegio, O. R., O'Connor, W., Sutterwala, F. S., and Flavell, R. A. (2008). Crucial role for the Nalp3 inflammasome in the immunostimulatory properties of aluminium adjuvants. *Nature* **453,** 1122.

Fink, S. L., and Cookson, B. T. (2005). Apoptosis, pyroptosis, and necrosis: mechanistic description of dead and dying eukaryotic cells. *Infect. Immun.* **73,** 1907.

Forsyth, R. A., Haselbeck, R. J., Ohlsen, K. L., Yamamoto, R. T., Xu, H., Trawick, J. D., Wall, D., Wang, L., Brown-Driver, V., Froelich, J. M., C, K. G., King, P., *et al.* (2002). A genome-wide strategy for the identification of essential genes in Staphylococcus aureus. *Mol. Microbiol.* **43,** 1387.

Franchi, L., and Nunez, G. (2010). AIM2 joins the gang of microbial sensors. *Cell Host Microbe* **7,** 340.

Franchi, L., Kanneganti, T. D., Dubyak, G. R., and Nunez, G. (2007). Differential requirement of P2X7 receptor and intracellular K+ for caspase-1 activation induced by intracellular and extracellular bacteria. *J. Biol. Chem.* **282,** 18810.

French, C. T., Lao, P., Loraine, A. E., Matthews, B. T., Yu, H., and Dybvig, K. (2008). Large-scale transposon mutagenesis of Mycoplasma pulmonis. *Mol. Microbiol.* **69,** 67.

Gilchrist, M., Thorsson, V., Li, B., Rust, A. G., Korb, M., Roach, J. C., Kennedy, K., Hai, T., Bolouri, H., and Aderem, A. (2006). Systems biology approaches identify ATF3 as a negative regulator of Toll-like receptor 4. *Nature* **441,** 173.

Glass, J. I., Assad-Garcia, N., Alperovich, N., Yooseph, S., Lewis, M. R., Maruf, M., Hutchison, C. A., 3rd, Smith, H. O., and Venter, J. C. (2006). Essential genes of a minimal bacterium. *Proc. Natl. Acad. Sci. USA* **103,** 425.

Gouin, E., Welch, M. D., and Cossart, P. (2005). Actin-based motility of intracellular pathogens. *Curr. Opin. Microbiol.* **8,** 35.

Gravekamp, C., and Paterson, Y. (2010). Harnessing Listeria monocytogenes to target tumors. *Cancer Biol. Ther.* **9,** 257–265.

Hamon, M., Bierne, H., and Cossart, P. (2006). Listeria monocytogenes: a multifaceted model. *Nat. Rev. Microbiol.* **4,** 423.

Harty, J. T., and Badovinac, V. P. (2008). Shaping and reshaping CD8+ T-cell memory. *Nat. Rev. Immunol.* **8,** 107.

Harty, J. T., and White, D. (1999). A knockout approach to understanding CD8+ cell effector mechanisms in adaptive immunity to Listeria monocytogenes. *Immunobiology* **201,** 196.

Harty, J. T., Tvinnereim, A. R., and White, D. W. (2000). CD8+ T cell effector mechanisms in resistance to infection. *Annu. Rev. Immunol.* **18,** 275.

Hayashi, F., Smith, K. D., Ozinsky, A., Hawn, T. R., Yi, E. C., Goodlett, D. R., Eng, J. K., Akira, S., Underhill, D. M., and Aderem, A. (2001). The innate immune response to bacterial flagellin is mediated by Toll-like receptor 5. *Nature* **410,** 1099.

Hu, D. L., Narita, K., Hyodo, M., Hayakawa, Y., Nakane, A., and Karaolis, D. K. (2009). c-di-GMP as a vaccine adjuvant enhances protection against systemic methicillin-resistant Staphylococcus aureus (MRSA) infection. *Vaccine* **27,** 4867.

Ichinohe, T., Lee, H. K., Ogura, Y., Flavell, R., and Iwasaki, A. (2009). Inflammasome recognition of influenza virus is essential for adaptive immune responses. *J. Exp. Med.* **206,** 79.

Janot, L., Secher, T., Torres, D., Maillet, I., Pfeilschifter, J., Quesniaux, V. F., Landmann, R., Ryffel, B., and Erard, F. (2008). CD14 works with toll-like receptor 2 to contribute to recogntion and control of Listeria monocytogenes infection. *J. Infect. Dis.* **198,** 115.

Jin, L., Hill, K. K., Filak, H., Mogan, J., Knowles, H., Zhang, B., Perraud, A. L., Cambier, J. C., and Lenz, L. L. (2011). MPYS is required for IFN response factor 3 activation and type 1 IFN production in the response of cultured phagocytes to bacterial second messengers cyclic-di-AMP and cyclic-di-GMP. *J. Immunol.* **187,** 2595.

Kagan, J. C., Su, T., Horng, T., Chow, A., Akira, S., and Medzhitov, R. (2008). TRAM couples endocytosis of Toll-like receptor 4 to the induction of interferon-beta. *Nat. Immunol.* **9,** 361.

Karaolis, D. K., Means, T. K., Yang, D., Takahashi, M., Yoshimura, T., Muraille, E., Philpott, D., Schroeder, J. T., Hyodo, M., Hayakawa, Y., Talbot, B. G., Brouillette, E., *et al.* (2007). Bacterial c-di-GMP is an immunostimulatory molecule. *J. Immunol.* **178,** 2171.

Kawai, T., and Akira, S. (2010). The role of pattern-recognition receptors in innate immunity: update on Toll-like receptors. *Nat. Immunol.* **11,** 373.

Kim, S., Bauernfeind, F., Ablasser, A., Hartmann, G., Fitzgerald, K. A., Latz, E., and Hornung, V. (2010). Listeria monocytogenes is sensed by the NLRP3 and AIM2 inflammasome. *Eur. J. Immunol.* **40,** 1545.

Kobayashi, K. S., Chamaillard, M., Ogura, Y., Henegariu, O., Inohara, N., Nunez, G., and Flavell, R. A. (2005). Nod2-dependent regulation of innate and adaptive immunity in the intestinal tract. *Science* **307,** 731.

Korn, T., Bettelli, E., Oukka, M., and Kuchroo, V. K. (2009). IL-17 and Th17 Cells. *Annu. Rev. Immunol.* **27,** 485.

Kumar, H., Kumagai, Y., Tsuchida, T., Koenig, P. A., Satoh, T., Guo, Z., Jang, M. H., Saitoh, T., Akira, S., and Kawai, T. (2009). Involvement of the NLRP3 inflammasome in innate and humoral adaptive immune responses to fungal beta-glucan. *J. Immunol.* **183,** 8061.

Lane, F. C., and Unanue, E. R. (1972). Requirement of thymus (T) lymphocytes for resistance to listeriosis. *J. Exp. Med.* **135,** 1104.

Lauvau, G., Vijh, S., Kong, P., Horng, T., Kerksiek, K., Serbina, N., Tuma, R. A., and Pamer, E. G. (2001). Priming of memory by not effector CD8 T cells by a killed bacterial vaccine. *Science* **294,** 1735.

Leber, J. H., Crimmins, G. T., Raghavan, S., Meyer, M. P., Cox, J. S., and Portnoy, D. A. (2008). Distinct TLR- and NLR-mediated transcriptional responses to an intracellular pathogen. *PLoS Pathog.* **4,** e6.

Lewinson, O., Adler, J., Sigal, N., and Bibi, E. (2006). Promiscuity in multidrug recognition and transport: the bacterial MFS Mdr transporters. *Mol. Microbiol.* **61,** 277.

Libanova, R., Ebensen, T., Schulze, K., Bruhn, D., Norder, M., Yevsa, T., Morr, M., and Guzman, C. A. (2010). The member of the cyclic di-nucleotide family bis-(3′, 5′)-cyclic dimeric inosine monophosphate exerts potent activity as mucosal adjuvant. *Vaccine* **28,** 2249.

Mackaness, M. (1962). Cellular resistance to infection. *J. Exp. Med.* **116,** 381.

Mackaness, G. B. (1964). The immunological basis of acquired cellular resistance. *J. Exp. Med.* **120,** 105.

Madhun, A. S., Haaheim, L. R., Nostbakken, J. K., Ebensen, T., Chichester, J., Yusibov, V., Guzman, C. A., and Cox, R. J. (2011). Intranasal c-di-GMP-adjuvanted plant-derived H5 influenza vaccine induces multifunctional Th1 CD4+ cells and strong mucosal and systemic antibody responses in mice. *Vaccine* **29,** 4973.

Mariathasan, S., Weiss, D. S., Newton, K., McBride, J., O'Rourke, K., Roose-Girma, M., Lee, W. P., Weinrauch, Y., Monack, D. M., and Dixit, V. M. (2006). Cryopyrin activates the inflammasome in response to toxins and ATP. *Nature* **440,** 228.

Martinon, F., Mayor, A., and Tschopp, J. (2009). The inflammasomes: guardians of the body. *Annu. Rev. Immunol.* **27,** 229.

Mbow, M. L., De Gregorio, E., Valiante, N. M., and Rappuoli, R. (2010). New adjuvants for human vaccines. *Curr. Opin. Immunol.* **22,** 411.

McCaffrey, R. L., Fawcett, P., O'Riordan, M., Lee, K. D., Havell, E. A., Brown, P. O., and Portnoy, D. A. (2004). A specific gene expression program triggered by Gram-positive bacteria in the cytosol. *Proc. Natl. Acad. Sci. USA* **101,** 11386.

McWhirter, S. M., Barbalat, R., Monroe, K. M., Fontana, M. F., Hyodo, M., Joncker, N. T., Ishii, K. J., Akira, S., Colonna, M., Chen, Z. J., Fitzgerald, K. A., Hayakawa, Y., *et al.* (2009). A host type 1 interferon response is induced by cytosolic sensing of the bacterial second messenger cyclic-di-GMP. *J. Exp. Med.* **206,** 1899–1911.

Meng, G., Zhang, F., Fuss, I., Kitani, A., and Strober, W. (2009). A mutation in the Nlrp2 gene causing inflammasome hyperactivation potentiates Th17 cell-dominant immune responses. *Immunity* **30,** 860.

Miao, E. A., Leaf, I. A., Treuting, P. M., Mao, D. P., Dors, M., Sarkar, A., Warren, S. E., Wewers, M. D., and Aderem, A. (2010). Caspase-1-induced pyroptosis is an innate immune effector mechanism against intracellular bacteria. *Nat. Immunol.* **11,** 1136.

North, R. J. (1973). Cellular mediators of anti-Listeria immunity as an enlarged population of short lived, replicating T cells. Kinetics of their production. *J. Exp. Med.* **138,** 342.

Ogunniyi, A. D., Paton, J. C., Kirby, A. C., McCullers, J. A., Cook, J., Hyodo, M., Hayakawa, Y., and Karaolis, D. K. (2008). c-di-GMP is an effective immunomodulator and vaccine adjuvant against pneumococcal infection. *Vaccine* **26,** 4676.

Orgun, N. N., and Way, S. S. (2008). A critical role for phospholipase C in protective immunity conferred by listeriolysin O-deficient Listeria monocytogenes. *Microb. Pathog.* **44,** 159.

O'Riordan, M., Yi, C. H., Gonzales, R., Lee, K. D., and Portnoy, D. A. (2002). Innate recognition of bacteria by a macrophage cytosolic surveillance pathway. *Proc. Natl. Acad. Sci. USA* **99,** 13861.

Pamer, E. G. (2004). Immune respsones to Listeria monocytogenes. *Nat. Rev. Immunol.* **4,** 812.

Persson, J., and Vance, R. E. (2007). Genetics-squared: combining host and pathogen genetics in the analysis of innate immunity and bacterial virulence. *Immunogenetics* **59,** 761.

Portnoy, D. A., Auerbuch, V., and Glomski, I. J. (2002). The cell biology of Listeria monocytogenes infection: the intersection of bacterial pathogenesis and cell-mediated immunity. *J. Cell Biol.* **158,** 409.

Quillin, S. J., Schwartz, K. T., and Leber, J. H. (2011). The novel Listeria monocytogenes bile sensor BrtA controls expression of the cholic acid efflux pump MdrT. *Mol. Microbiol.* **81,** 129.

Rae, C. S., Geissler, A., Adamson, P. C., and Portnoy, D. A. (2011). Mutations of the Listeria monocytogenes peptidoglycan N-deacetylase result in enhanced lysozyme sensitivity, bacteriolysis, and hyperinduction of innate immune pathways. *Infect. Immun.* **79,** 3596.

Rao, F., See, R. Y., Zhang, D., Toh, D. C., Ji, Q., and Liang, Z. X. (2010). YybT is a signaling protein that contains a cyclic dinucleotide phosphodiesterase domain and a GGDEF domain with ATPase activity. *J. Biol. Chem.* **285,** 473.

Romling, U. (2008). Great times for small molecules: c-di-AMP, a second messenger candidate in Bacteria and Archaea. *Sci. Signal.* **1,** pe39.

Sauer, J. D., Witte, C. E., Zemansky, J., Hanson, B., Lauer, P., and Portnoy, D. A. (2010). Listeria monocytogenes triggers AIM2-mediated pyroptosis upon infrequent bacteriolysis in the macrophage cytosol. *Cell Host Microbe* **7,** 412.

Sauer, J. D., Pereyre, S., Archer, K. A., Burke, T. P., Hanson, B., Lauer, P., and Portnoy, D. A. (2011a). Listeria monocytogenes engineered to activate the Nlrc4 inflammasome are severely attenuated and are poor inducers of protective immunity. *Proc. Natl. Acad. Sci. USA* **108,** 12419–12424.

Sauer, J. D., Sotelo-Troha, K., von Moltke, J., Monroe, K. M., Rae, C. S., Brubaker, S. W., Hyodo, M., Hayakawa, Y., Woodward, J. J., Portnoy, D. A., and Vance, R. E. (2011b). The N-ethyl-N-nitrosourea-induced Goldenticket mouse mutant reveals an essential function of Sting in the in vivo interferon response to Listeria and cyclic dinucleotides. *Infect. Immun.* **79,** 688.

Schenten, D., and Medzhitov, R. (2011). The control of adaptive immune responses by the innate immune system. *Adv. Immunol.* **109,** 87.

Schnupf, P., and Portnoy, D. A. (2007). Listeriolysin O: a phagosome-specific lysin. *Microbes Infect.* **9,** 1176.

Seubert, A., Calabro, S., Santini, L., Galli, B., Genovese, A., Valentini, S., Aprea, S., Colaprico, A., D'Oro, U., Giuliani, M. M., Pallaoro, M., Pizza, M., *et al.* (2011). Adjuvanticity of the oil-in-water emulsion MF59 is independent of Nlrp3 inflammasome but requires the adaptor protein MyD88. *Proc. Natl. Acad. Sci. USA* **108,** 11169.

Shen, A., and Higgins, D. E. (2006). The MogR transcriptional repressor regulates nonhierarchal expression of flagellar motility genes and virulence in Listera monocytogenes. *PLoS Pathog.* **2,** e30.

Song, J. H., Ko, K. S., Lee, J. Y., Baek, J. Y., Oh, W. S., Yoon, H. S., Jeong, J. Y., and Chun, J. (2005). Indentification of essential genes in Streptococcus pneumoniae by allelic replacement mutagenesis. *Mol. Cells* **19,** 365.

Stetson, D. B., and Medzhitov, R. (2006). Type 1 interferons in host defense. *Immunity* **24,** 93.

Tabeta, K., Hoebe, K., Janssen, E. M., Du, X., Georgel, P., Crozat, K., Mudd, S., Mann, N., Sovath, S., Goode, J., Shamel, L., Herskovits, A. A., *et al.* (2006). The Unc93b1 mutation 3d disrupts exogenous antigen presentation and signaling via Toll-like receptors 3, 7 and 9. *Nat. Immunol.* **7,** 156.

Tilney, L. G., and Portnoy, D. A. (1989). Actin filaments and the growth, movement, and spread of the intracellular bacterial parasite, Listeria monocytogenes. *J. Cell Biol.* **109,** 1597.

Torres, D., Barrier, M., Bihl, F., Quesniaux, V. J., Maillet, I., Akira, S., Ryffel, B., and Erard, F. (2004). Toll-like receptor 2 is required for optimal control of Listeria monocytogenes infection. *Infect. Immun.* **72,** 2131.

Travassos, L., Girardin, S., Philpott, D., Blanot, D., Nahori, M., Werts, C., and Boneca, I. (2004). Toll-like receptor 2-dependent bacterial sensing does not occur via peptidoglycan recognition. *EMBO Rep.* **5,** 1000.

Uematsu, S., Jang, M. H., Chevrier, N., Guo, Z., Kumagai, Y., Yamamoto, M., Kato, H., Sougawa, N., Matsui, H., Kuwata, H., Hemmi, H., Coban, C., *et al.* (2006). Detection of pathogenic intestinal bacteria by Toll-like receptor 5 on intestinal CD11c+ lamina propria cells. *Nat. Immunol.* **7,** 868.

Unanue, E. R. (1997). Studies in listeriosis show the strong symbiosis between the innate cellular system and the T-cell response. *Immunol. Rev.* **158,** 11.

Vance, R. E., Isberg, R. R., and Portnoy, D. A. (2009). Patterns of pathogenesis: discrimination of pathogenic and nonpathogenic microbes by the innate immune system. *Cell Host Microbe* **6,** 10.

von Koenig, C. H. W., Finger, H., and Hof, H. (1982). Failure of killed Listeria monocytogenes vaccine to produce protective immunity. *Nature* **297,** 233.

Warren, S. E., Mao, D. P., Rodriguez, A. E., Miao, E. A., and Aderem, A. (2008). Multiple Nod-like receptors activate caspase 1 during Listeria monocytogenes infection. *J. Immunol.* **180,** 7558.

Warren, S. E., Armstrong, A., Hamilton, M. K., Mao, D. P., Leaf, I. A., Miao, E. A., and Aderem, A. (2010). Cutting edge: Cytosolic bacterial DNA activates the inflammasome via Aim2. *J. Immunol.* **185,** 818–821.

Watanabe, H., Gehrke, S., Contassot, E., Roques, S., Tschopp, J., Friedmann, P. S., French, L. E., and Gaide, O. (2008). Danger sensing throught the inflammasome acts as a master switch between tolerance and sensitization. *J. Immunol.* **180,** 5826.

Way, S. S., Kollmann, T. R., Hajjar, A. M., and Wilson, C. B. (2003). Cutting edge: protective cell-mediated immunity to Listeria monocytogenes in the absence of myeloid differntiation factor 88. *J. Immunol.* **171,** 533.

Witte, G., Hartung, S., Buttner, K., and Hopfner, K. P. (2008). Structural biochemistry of a bacterial checkpoint protein reveals diadenylate cyclase activity regulated by DNA recombination intermediates. *Mol. Cell* **30,** 167.

Woodward, J. J., Iavarone, A. T., and Portnoy, D. A. (2010). c-di-AMP secreted by intracellular Listeria monocytogenes activates a host type 1 interferon response. *Science* **328,** 1703–1705.

Wu, J., Fernandes-Alnemri, T., and Alnemri, E. S. (2010). Involvement of the AIM2, NLRC4, and NLRP3 inflammasomes in caspase-1 activation by Listeria monocytogenes. *J. Clin. Immunol.* **30,** 693–702.

Zemansky, J., Kline, B. C., Woodward, J. J., Leber, J. H., Marquis, H., and Portnoy, D. A. (2009). Development of a mariner-based transposon and identification of Listeria monocytogenes determinants, including the peptidyl-prolyl isomerase PrsA2, that contribute to its hemolytic phenotype. *J. Bacteriol.* **191,** 3950.

CHAPTER 9

Mechanisms and Immunological Effects of Apoptosis Caused by *Listeria Monocytogenes*

Javier A. Carrero and **Emil R. Unanue**

Contents

Abstract

Infection with *Listeria monocytogenes* shows an early stage of lymphocyte apoptosis. This is an obligatory stage the extent of which depends on infective dose. Lymphocyte apoptosis occurs early and is rapidly superseded, yet it has a strong biological

Department of Pathology and Immunology, Washington University School of Medicine, St. Louis, Missouri, USA

Advances in Immunology, Volume 113
ISSN 0065-2776, DOI: 10.1016/B978-0-12-394590-7.00001-4

consequence. The immunological effect of lymphocyte apoptosis following infection is increased susceptibility to *L. monocytogenes* infection due, in part, to upregulation of IL-10 on macrophages and DC. Lymphocyte apoptosis is dependent on bacterial expression of the pore-forming toxin listeriolysin O (LLO). Also, purified LLO can lead to the induction of death pathways similar to infection, demonstrating that it is a killer agent generated by *L. monocytogenes*. Signaling through the type I interferon receptor potentiates cell death induced by the bacteria or LLO. Infection with *L. monocytogenes* also causes death of phagocytic cells, the nature and significance of which is not clear at present. Infection with *L. monocytogenes* is a tractable model to examine pathogen-induced cell death pathways and their possible immunological consequences in multiple cell types following infection.

1. INTRODUCTION: APOPTOSIS FOLLOWING INFECTION WITH *L. MONOCYTOGENES*

A long-standing finding during *L. monocytogenes* infection of mice was the rapid, synchronous, and extensive depletion of lymphocytes surrounding the periarteriolar lymphoid sheaths (PALS) (Mandel and Cheers, 1980). Regardless of a mouse strain's susceptibility, depletion occurred 1–3 days postinfection. Neither splenic migration nor adrenal hormones were involved in this depletion (Chan and Cheers, 1982). Subsequent examination explained the lesions as caused by lymphocyte death. The death of T lymphocytes in the PALS induced by *L. monocytogenes* was apoptotic in nature and preceded antigen-specific activation (Merrick *et al.*, 1997). Apoptotic lesions were detected in the spleens, lymph nodes, livers, and brains of *L. monocytogenes*-infected mice (Merrick *et al.*, 1997; Rogers *et al.*, 1996; Schluter *et al.*, 1998). The splenic and hepatic apoptotic lesions were carefully evaluated, and all strains of conventional mice examined contained them following intraperitoneal or intravenous infection. The only distinction among normal mice was the median lethal dose of a particular strain. More initial inoculum was required to obtain equivalent lesions in an infection-resistant strain, such as C57BL/6, than a susceptible strain, such as BALB/c. Route of infection had no effect on the magnitude or timing of splenic or hepatic apoptotic lesions. Neuronal apoptosis was found after intracerebral infection. To our knowledge, no one has examined the Peyer's patches, intraepithelial lymphocytes, lamina propria, or mesenteric lymph nodes for signs of cell death following an oral infection with *L. monocytogenes*, the natural route of infection.

The use of terminal deoxynucleotidyl transferase dUTP nick end labeling (TUNEL) and electron microscopy (EM) revealed that the cell death taking place in the spleen, liver, and lymph nodes was apoptotic in

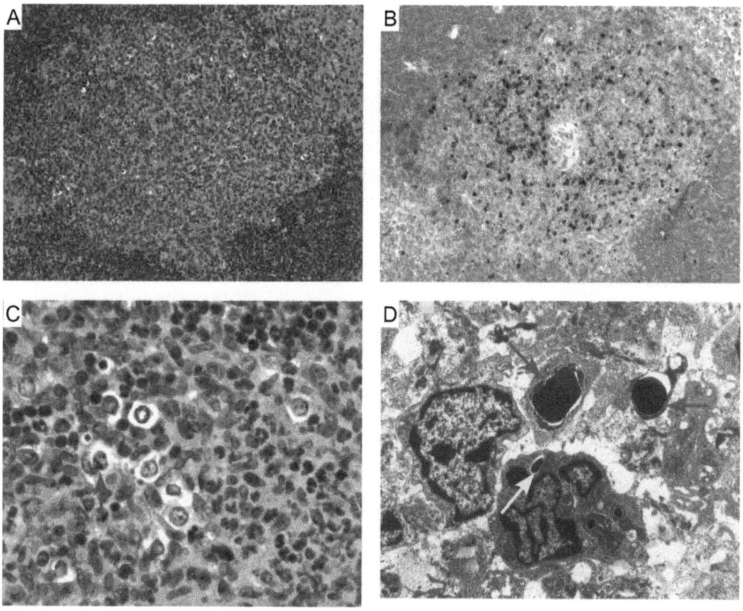

FIGURE 9.1 Histological analysis of spleens following infection with *L. monocytogenes* (A–C). C57BL/6 mice were infected with 10^5 CFU of *L. monocytogenes* EGD strain for 2 days. Spleens were fixed and embedded and then stained by hematoxylin and eosin (A, C) or by TUNEL (B). (C) The red arrow shows an apoptotic cell that is contained inside a phagocytic vacuole. (D) C.B-17 mice were infected with 10^4 CFU of *L. monocytogenes* EGD strain for 48 h. Spleens were removed and processed for electron microscopy. Red arrows show apoptotic nuclei. The yellow arrow shows a bacterium inside a macrophage. (See Color Insert.)

nature. Figure 9.1 shows representative histological evaluation of the spleens of *L. monocytogenes*-infected mice. The earliest TUNEL$^+$ lymphocytes were detected after 24 h in spleens following intravenous infection and in popliteal lymph nodes following footpad infection (Merrick *et al.*, 1997). The peak of TUNEL$^+$ lymphocytes occurred at 48 h and was fully resolved by 96 h postinfection with no detectable apoptotic nuclei. The lymphocyte apoptotic stage was brief and rapidly superseded, yet it had biological consequences described below. Lymph node TUNEL$^+$ staining also peaked at 48 h postinfection and was localized to the deep cortex, again, tracking with the T cell zone. In the spleen, the zone of cell death was restricted to the white pulp, the T cell zone of the spleen. No increase in cell death was detected in the red pulp. In both spleens and lymph nodes, the size of the lesions depended on the infectious dose, with higher doses leading to larger lesions. In the case of spleen, more individual white pulp profiles were affected at higher infectious doses. Despite the enlargement of the lesion size, B cell regions appeared to be spared from apoptosis, but more detailed examination is needed to confirm this observation.

The presence of condensed nuclei and membrane blebbing was found by EM confirming that the lesions were apoptotic in nature. Importantly, the lymphocytes were not infected with *L. monocytogenes*, indicating that apoptosis was caused by a factor extrinsic to the dying cell. Throughout the infection, *L. monocytogenes* was found inside phagocytic cells, an observation that was confirmed by multiple studies using fluorescence microscopy and flow cytometry (Aoshi *et al.*, 2009; Muraille *et al.*, 2005; Neuenhahn *et al.*, 2006). Indeed, the major carriers of *L. monocytogenes* during the peak of apoptosis in the spleen at 48 h were macrophages and neutrophils. There was also cell death in the phagocytic lineages, but it involved necrotic profiles that either contained bacteria or had adjacent extracellular bacteria. The apoptotic nuclei of lymphocytes were found in close apposition to the necrotic profiles of phagocytes, suggesting that the dying phagocyte or the extracellular bacteria secreted an apoptogenic agent (Carrero *et al.*, 2006; Merrick *et al.*, 1997).

In the livers, apoptosis was detected in hepatocytes by 12–16 h following infection with a peak TUNEL^{+} staining after 24 h (Rogers *et al.*, 1996). Immunofluorescent staining by TUNEL and anti-*Listeria* antibodies showed that cell death colocalized with bacterial infection. Electron microscope studies detected infected hepatocytes with apoptotic nuclei. *In vitro* infection of purified hepatocytes also led to apoptosis as determined by nuclear condensation, DNA fragmentation, membrane blebbing, and lactate dehydrogenase (LDH) release 4–6 h following infection. Since hepatocyte cell death was not dependent on the leukocytes that infiltrated the initial lesion, apoptosis was replicated *ex vivo* by infecting purified primary hepatocytes. Therefore, unlike lymphocytes, direct infection of the hepatocyte was responsible for the induction of apoptosis. The early hepatic lesions were microabscesses rich in neutrophil infiltrates surrounded by TUNEL^{+} dying hepatocytes. Neutrophil depletion accelerated the appearance as well as increased the number of TUNEL^{+} hepatocytes, allowing clear visualization of cell death within 12 h. Apoptotic hepatocytes released chemoattractants for neutrophils, such as CXCL1, so that the death phase may also be important for recruitment of neutrophils and for control of the infection (Rogers *et al.*, 1996).

Intracerebral infection with *L. monocytogenes* led to apoptosis of neurons that was restricted to the hippocampal CA1 region, despite the presence of bacteria at other locations in the brain (Schluter *et al.*, 1998). Hippocampal lesions were TUNEL^{+} at day 3 postinfection, and apoptotic leukocytes were detected at days 3 and 5 postinfection in the ventricular lumen. Necrotic cell death was also evident in the plexus epithelium, ependymal layer, and brain parenchyma. Little is known about the mechanisms or effects of neuron-specific cell death during *L. monocytogenes* infection. It would be interesting to understand why certain neuroanatomical locations are susceptible to apoptosis or necrotic death.

2. MODULATION OF *IN VIVO* APOPTOTIC LESION FORMATION FOLLOWING INFECTION

We studied the lymphocyte apoptosis stage of infection in many different strains of mice. Additionally, treatments with monoclonal antibodies specific to various cytokines and cytokine receptors were tested. Table 9.1 shows all the manipulations that were examined and their effect on cell death. Almost all the treatments that increased apoptosis following infection were essential early innate immune effectors that were either blocked or deleted. Depletion of neutrophils, blockade of tumor necrosis factor-α (TNF-α) with antibody or by genetic ablation of the TNF-α receptors, removal of most toll-like receptor signaling by deletion of *Myd88*, and removal of interferon-γ (IFN-γ) receptor (IFN-γR) signaling, all permitted more bacterial growth and increased apoptosis in spleens and livers. Most of the known host-derived pathways for the induction of apoptosis were not involved in the development of the apoptotic lesions following infection with *L. monocytogenes*. Mice deficient in Fas/FasL signaling, TNF-RI signaling, and perforin all had apoptotic lesions of comparable magnitude and abundance. Infection of Bcl-2 transgenic mice or mice treated with the pan-caspase inhibitor z-VAD-FMK still contained the apoptotic lesions. The three host manipulations shown to reduce apoptosis following infection were TNF-related apoptosis-inducing ligand (TRAIL) deficiency/ soluble DR5 (TRAIL antagonist), type I interferon receptor deficiency (IFN-αβR$^{-/-}$), and granzymes (gzms) deficiency (Auerbuch *et al.*, 2004; Carrero *et al.*, 2004b, 2008; O'Connell *et al.*, 2004; Zheng *et al.*, 2004). One manipulation, genetic deletion of the liver X receptor (LXR), permitted increased apoptosis in the macrophage that correlated with increased bacterial growth (Joseph *et al.*, 2004).

The induction of apoptosis required live infection with *L. monocytogenes* since heat-killed bacteria did not induce cell death (Merrick *et al.*, 1997). Apoptosis was absent following a secondary challenge or treatment with anti-LLO antibodies, which neutralized *L. monocytogenes* infection (Edelson and Unanue, 2001; Edelson *et al.*, 1999). Neutralization of LLO reduced the number of microbes in the spleen and liver, so the reduction in apoptosis was correlated with a decrease in bacterial burden.

The correlation of infectious dose with the extent of apoptotic lesions implies that a bacterial product may induce or potentiate cell death pathways. We tested *L. monocytogenes* strains that were deficient in various virulence factors, including LLO, internalins, and phospholipases

TABLE 9.1 Effect of different manipulations on the lymphocyte apoptosis detected following *L. monocytogenes* infection

Increase in leukocyte death	Same degree of leukocyte death	Leukocyte death decreased or absent
Anti-Ly6C/G: RB6.8C5	Irrelevant antibody L2309	Heat-killed *L. monocytogenes*
Anti-TNF-α: TN319.2	Anti-IFN-γ: H22	Secondary *L. monocytogenes* challenge
IFN-αβR$^{-/-}$ × IFN-γ R$^{-/-}$ mice	Anti-IL-1R: JAMA 147	Anti-LLO: A4–8
IFN-γ$^{-/-}$ mice	Anti-IL-12: Tosh/Red T	Soluble DR5 (TRAIL antagonist)
TNF-RI$^{-/-}$	BL6/lpr mice	TRAIL$^{-/-}$ mice
TNF-RI$^{-/-}$ × TNF-RII$^{-/-}$ mice	3A9 TCR transgenic mice	IFN-αβR$^{-/-}$ mice
MyD88$^{-/-}$ mice	TNF-RII$^{-/-}$ mice	Granzyme A$^{-/-}$ × B cluster$^{-/-}$ mice
LXR-αβ$^{-/-}$ mice	Perforin$^{-/-}$ mice	Surface-tethered LLO strain (sLLO)
IL-6$^{-/-}$ mice	Phospholipase-deficient *Listeria*	RAG$^{-/-}$ mice
	IL-10$^{-/-}$ mice	SCID mice
	Aminoguanidine	
	Internalin-deficient *L. monocytogenes*	

Citations are included in the text.

(Merrick *et al.*, 1997; our unpublished observations). The only strain that did not induce apoptosis *in vivo* was the LLO-deficient strain.

The induction of lymphocytes apoptosis was not dependent on antigenic specificity (Jiang *et al.*, 2003). TCR transgenic mice that only responded to a hen egg lysozyme epitope (3A9) still contained apoptotic lesions. In contrast, antigen-specific lymphocytes proliferated through the apoptosis induced by *L. monocytogenes*. CFSE-labeled lymphocytic choriomeningitis virus glycoprotein 33 (LCMV-gp33)-specific CD8 T cells were detected in the PALS of mice following adoptive transfer into normal recipients. The gp33-reactive CD8 T cells became TUNEL^{+} following infection with either a normal strain of *L. monocytogenes* or a strain harboring a transgene for the LCMV-gp33 protein, but some of the antigen specific cells proliferated in response to the infection. In sum and in agreement with the results following infection of the 3A9 TCR transgenic mouse, the induction of apoptosis was antigen independent.

3. INDUCTION OF LYMPHOCYTE APOPTOSIS BY LLO

The results using monoclonal antibodies against LLO and infection with LLO-deficient microbes, which resulted in reduced or absent apoptotic lesions, pointed to LLO as the causative molecule. LLO is a member of the cholesterol-dependent cytolysin/membrane attack complex/perforin (CDC/MACPF) superfamily of toxins (Gilbert, 2010; Heuck *et al.*, 2010; Rosado *et al.*, 2007). The role of LLO in the virulence of *L. monocytogenes* infection has been reviewed extensively (see Kayal and Charbit, 2006; Schnupf and Portnoy, 2007). Briefly, endocytosed *L. monocytogenes* required LLO to escape the endosome/phagosome of the infected cell. Bacteria trapped in phagosomes were efficiently killed even in the absence of any inflammatory activation. In addition to its role in promoting the survival of *L. monocytogenes*, LLO had multiple effects on different cell types (Kayal and Charbit, 2006). LLO caused transient calcium fluxes at the cell surface, induced MAP kinase activation, and was responsible for a type I interferon cascade in infected cells (O'Riordan *et al.*, 2002; Tang *et al.*, 1996; Wadsworth and Goldfine, 1999). The activity of LLO was dependent on pH and the reductive potential of the vesicular compartment (Glomski *et al.*, 2002; Singh *et al.*, 2008).

LLO had been used as a substitute for perforin to deliver exogenous purified gzmB into target cells. LLO delivery of gzmB was independent of pore formation on the cell surface. LLO had two effects on gzmB, it increased the uptake of the protease by target cells and caused it to transit from the cytosol to the nucleus through an undefined mechanism. While the focus of this work was to determine the mechanism of perforin activity, it also demonstrated that LLO and other members of the CDC family could have activities in cells that mimic perforin and can lead to autologous apoptosis via alteration of gzmB localization inside the cell (Browne *et al.*, 1999).

Treatment of cultured lymphocytes with purified recombinant LLO induced apoptosis (Carrero *et al.*, 2004a). The amount of LLO required to induce lymphocyte apoptosis ranged from 0.4 to 4 nM, whereas necrotic killing of cells ranged from 20 to 40 nM. Importantly, LLO-induced apoptosis was dependent on the activation state of the T cells. Rapidly dividing lymphocytes were susceptible to apoptosis, while resting lymphocytes were resistant.

Treatment with type I interferon primed resting lymphocytes to undergo apoptosis induced by LLO (Carrero *et al.*, 2004b). Type I interferon has pleiotropic effects on multiple cell types, so there are many changes that could take place on lymphocytes to increase their susceptibility to cell death (Honda *et al.*, 2006). Possible changes include alteration of membrane composition (Bougnoux *et al.*, 1985; Zwaferink *et al.*, 2008) and activation of proapoptotic enzymes, such as caspases (Chen *et al.*, 2001).

The proapoptogenic effect of type I interferon on lymphocytes negatively influences the response to *L. monocytogenes* following infection of mice (Carrero *et al.*, 2004b, 2006, see Section 5).

Lymphocyte apoptosis occurred in two phases, a fast gzm-dependent pathway and a slow unresolved pathway. The fast phase of cell death proceeded through activation of caspase-3, -6, and -9 by intracellular gzmB (Carrero *et al.*, 2008). Fast apoptosis was inhibited by z-VAD-FMK or by genetic ablation of gzms. The slow phase of apoptosis was not inhibited by z-VAD-FMK or by deletion of gzms. Neither fast nor slow apoptotic pathways were calcium dependent, as determined by removal of calcium from the medium, calcium chelation, and calpain inhibition.

Exposure of phosphatidylserine, depolarization of the mitochondria, and internucleosomal DNA fragmentation was evident in both fast and slow apoptosis. Caspase activation was detected as early as 30 min following treatment with LLO, with peak activation after 1 h. Phosphatidylserine exposure was detected within 1 h and climaxed between 2 and 4 h posttreatment with LLO. Mitochondrial depolarization was evident by 2 h and was maximal by 4 h. DNA fragmentation into internucleosomal fragments of ~200 bp was found after 12 h by both TUNEL-staining and agarose gel electrophoresis. Neutralization of phagosomal acidity using chloroquine prevented the rapid apoptosis and reduced the slow apoptosis (Carrero *et al.*, 2008). The pH-dependent enhancement of LLO activity likely allows it to compromise the endosomal/phagosomal compartments, causing the release of their contents into the cytosol.

The presence of gzms in lymphocytes was required for the induction of fast apoptosis. Cells died with slower kinetics when gzms were removed, possibly due to the release/activation of other proteases or the induction of a stress-response pathway. One conundrum is that gzms are stored in functionally specialized lytic granules (Masson and Tschopp, 1987). It is unknown how extracellular LLO entered the cell and caused the activation of an intracellular gzms store. LLO may enter by endocytosis and cause aberrant fusion of endosomal compartments with the lytic granules, leading to translocation of gzms into the cytosol. Alternatively, gzms sequestration inside the cell may not be all-or-none, and some gzms may be found in recycling endosomes that fuse with LLO-bearing endocytic compartments. It would be interesting to dissect the localization of LLO inside cells and further examine the slow phase of cell death to determine the different ways that LLO can kill a cell.

Attempting to conclusively prove that LLO is a lymphocyte apoptotogenic agent *in vivo* is confounded by the obligate requirement of LLO expression for *L. monocytogenes* virulence in mice (Gaillard *et al.*, 1986; Portnoy *et al.*, 1988). Injection of purified LLO into the footpads of mice led to $TUNEL^+$ cells in the peripheral cortex and paracortex of the draining popliteal lymph node, but not the more distal inguinal lymph node

(Carrero *et al.*, 2004a). This demonstrated that LLO alone could induce all the parameters of apoptosis found after infection with *L. monocytogenes* in the footpad.

In order to determine the causal relationship of LLO to the induction of apoptosis in the context of live infection, a strain of *L. monocytogenes* with LLO tethered to the cell wall was engineered, rendering it a hyposecretor (Carrero *et al.*, 2009). The surface LLO (sLLO) strain behaved normally in all *in vitro* assays. It infected cells, grew at normal rates, exited from the phagosome to the cytosol, and spread to adjacent cells. Despite the normal *in vitro* phenotype, sLLO was attenuated *in vivo*. The LLO expressed by sLLO was still functional *in vivo* because treatment with anti-LLO antibodies reduced infectivity (Edelson *et al.*, 1999). During infection, *L. monocytogenes* was mostly intracellular, as determined by selective susceptibility to cell-permeable antibiotics (Glomski *et al.*, 2003). Treatment with antineutrophil antibodies has shown that there was a component of the infection that was extracellular (Conlan and North, 1994; Rogers and Unanue, 1993). The sLLO strain was sensitive to depletion of neutrophils, suggesting that, like wild-type *L. monocytogenes*, it had an extracellular component to its infection (Carrero *et al.*, 2009; Rogers and Unanue, 1993). Even after adjusting the input doses of wild type and sLLO bacteria to obtain equivalent output colony counts *in vivo*, there was reduced apoptosis in the spleen. This data is suggestive for a role for secreted extracellular LLO in the induction of apoptosis, but more work needs to be done. In particular, quantification of *in vivo* LLO production and determination of the number of extracellular microbes during infection need to be carried out.

4. INDUCTION OF CELL DEATH IN DENDRITIC CELLS OR MACROPHAGES FOLLOWING INFECTION WITH *L. MONOCYTOGENES* OR TREATMENT WITH LLO

Macrophages and DC are the first carriers of *L. monocytogenes* following a systemic infection (Aoshi *et al.*, 2009; Muraille *et al.*, 2005; Neuenhahn *et al.*, 2006). Their fate following infection is important because of their role in the containment of the bacteria as well as the activation of innate and adaptive immunity. Infection of the DC line CB1 or bone marrow-derived dendritic cells (BMDC) with *L. monocytogenes* led to apoptosis in 4–6 h (Guzman *et al.*, 1996). The induction of cell death was dependent on bacterial expression of LLO. Treatment with exogenous LLO also caused apoptosis within 8 h of treatment. The features of the DC cell-line apoptosis included internucleosomal DNA fragmentation, DNA condensation, and LDH release. Only DNA fragmentation was tested in granulocyte–macrophage colony-stimulating factor (GM-CSF)-derived BMDC. We have also treated GM-CSF BMDC with LLO and found activation of caspase-3, phosphatidylserine exposure, and depolarization of mitochondria, confirming that the cell death seen in DCs was apoptotic. Interestingly, DCs became infected very early following *L. monocytogenes* infection and trafficked from the marginal zone to the bridging areas and then into the PALS (Aoshi *et al.*, 2009). This migration was rapid and completed within 12 h of infection. After this time, there was a reduction in the number of detectable DCs, despite an increase in the number of bacteria. A possible role for *L. monocytogenes*-induced apoptosis in the reduction of DCs *in vivo* remains unexplored.

Results testing LLO and *L. monocytogenes*-induced cell death of macrophages are inconsistent and somewhat contradictory (Barsig and Kaufmann, 1997; Cervantes *et al.*, 2008; Joseph *et al.*, 2004; Sauer *et al.*, 2010; Zwaferink *et al.*, 2008). The observations of five independent groups will be summarized herein. The first study examined bone marrow-derived macrophages (BMM) generated with macrophage colony-stimulating factor (M-CSF) and found that cells died through a nonapoptotic cell death pathway following infection with *L. monocytogenes*. The authors were unable to define the form of cell death (Barsig and Kaufmann, 1997). In a second study, infection of the macrophage cell lines RAW264.7 and IC-21 with *L. monocytogenes* also caused cell death. The type of death did not have a mitochondrial depolarization involvement suggesting that it was not apoptotic in nature and was probably pyroptosis (Cervantes *et al.*, 2008). A third group treated BMM with type I interferon and this sensitized them to lysis by LLO. This study looked at immediate lytic death induced by LLO, not at programmed forms of cell death (Zwaferink *et al.*, 2008). A fourth study suggested that BMM died by pyroptosis (Sauer *et al.*, 2010). The fifth study was examination of *L. monocytogenes* susceptibility in LXR-$\alpha/\beta^{-/-}$ mice. The authors showed that RAW264.7 cells died by apoptosis (Joseph *et al.*, 2004). Enforced overexpression of LXR-β protected RAW264.7 from *L. monocytogenes*-induced apoptosis. This effect was mediated by LXR-β upregulation of SPα, an inhibitor of macrophage apoptosis.

In sum, examination of all the macrophage and DC cell death parameters induced by *L. monocytogenes* infection or LLO treatment needs to be performed. It will be important to determine if, under some inflammatory settings, macrophages can completely shut down apoptotic pathways, that is, by upregulating LXR/SPα, in order to favor a pyroptotic cell death. Since apoptosis is a negative regulator of the response to *L. monocytogenes* infection, LXR signaling may force macrophages to die by pyroptosis instead of apoptosis. This would lead to enhanced IL-1-dependent innate immune activation following infection (Carrero *et al.*, 2006; Joseph *et al.*, 2004). One simple test for this hypothesis would be to determine if *L. monocytogenes*-infected $LXR^{-/-}$ macrophages or mice produce reduced amount of active IL-1 when compared to wild-type counterparts.

5. INCREASED RESISTANCE TO INFECTION IN TYPE I INTERFERON-DEFICIENT MICE AND ITS RELATIONSHIP WITH CELL DEATH

IFN-$\alpha\beta R^{-/-}$ mice were more resistant to *L. monocytogenes* infection and had reduced apoptosis of splenic lymphocytes (Carrero *et al.*, 2004b; O'Connell *et al.*, 2004). This observation extended to two strains of *L. monocytogenes*, 10403S and EGD, and was found in three distinct genetic strains of mice (BALB/c, C57BL/6, and 129). This very surprising result contrasted with the protective effect of type I interferon on viral infections. These studies led to a number of investigations into the mechanisms underlying the detrimental effects of type I interferons on *L. monocytogenes* infection.

DCs and macrophages infected with *L. monocytogenes* induced expression of type I interferon and interferon-responsive genes *in vitro* (McCaffrey *et al.*, 2004; O'Riordan *et al.*, 2002). The cellular source of type I interferon following infection *in vivo* is not entirely clear, but $CD11b^{+}CD11c^{-}PDCA1^{-}B220^{-}$ macrophages and TNF/iNOS-producing dendritic cells (Tip-DC) were shown to produce the cytokine (Dresing *et al.*, 2010; Stockinger *et al.*, 2009). Whether other cells participate in the induction of type I interferon requires further studies. The upregulation of type I interferon genes by macrophages was dependent on the expression of LLO by *L. monocytogenes*. Enforced expression of LLO in *Bacillus subtilis* was sufficient to convert it from a noninducer to an inducer of type I interferon genes (McCaffrey *et al.*, 2004). The type I interferon produced *in vitro* during *L. monocytogenes* infection induced CD69 upregulation and increased the sensitivity of T cells to be activated by antigen (Feng *et al.*, 2005). This was compatible with work showing that preactivation of T cells occurred through type I interferon signaling (Sun *et al.*, 1998). *In vitro*, type I interferon-mediated T cell preactivation did not send the cells into cell cycle.

Reports that showed the preactivation of lymphocytes by type I interferon led us to investigate if this modulated host response to *L. monocytogenes* infection. In the absence of type I interferon signaling, there was reduced CD69 upregulation following infection, indicating an absence of preactivation (Auerbuch *et al.*, 2004; Carrero *et al.*, 2004b; O'Connell *et al.*, 2004). We proposed that the preactivation of lymphocytes by type I interferon sensitized them to the apoptogenic effect of LLO, with negative consequences on the handling of *L. monocytogenes* infection (Carrero *et al.*, 2004b; O'Connell *et al.*, 2004).

In addition to lymphocyte apoptosis, there was a type I interferon-dependent reduction of two $CD11b^{+}$ populations of cells following infection with *L. monocytogenes*. The reason for the depletion of the two $CD11b^{+}$ subsets, one a $CD11b^{int}$/Mac-3^{high}/$CD11c^{+}$ "Tip-DC" population and another a $CD11b^{high}$/Mac-$3^{int/high}$/$CD11c^{-}$ macrophage population, is undefined. Interestingly, the CD11b^{high}/Mac-3$^{int/high}$/CD11c^{-} population was a producer of TNF-α in IFN-αβR$^{-/-}$ mice. This would suggest that type I interferon-mediated cell death of macrophages during infection may limit the ability of wild-type mice to control infection with *L. monocytogenes* (Auerbuch *et al.*, 2004).

One component of the susceptibility to infection downstream of IFN-αβR signaling was IL-10 produced following the development of lymphocyte apoptotic bodies. An early production of IL-10 followed infection with *L. monocytogenes,* which was dependent on the presence of lymphocytes and intact IFN-αβR signaling. The only producers of IL-10 during the early innate response to *L. monocytogenes* infection were CD11b^{+} cells and CD11c^{+} cells. No IL-10 production was detected in CD19^{+} or CD3^{+} subsets. IL-10$^{-/-}$ mice were more resistant to *L. monocytogenes* infection despite having normal apoptotic lesions in the spleen (Carrero *et al.*, 2006; Dai *et al.*, 1997). These findings are compatible with a model wherein macrophages and DC engulf apoptotic lymphocytes and secrete IL-10 (Carrero and Unanue, 2006). In turn, IL-10 antagonizes IFN-γ signaling leading to increased susceptibility during early *L. monocytogenes* infection.

6. INCREASED RESISTANCE TO INFECTION IN LYMPHOCYTE-DEFICIENT MICE

During the early stage of infection, T and B-cell deficient mice (SCID and RAG$^{-/-}$) were more resistant to *L. monocytogenes* than normal mice. Yet, such mice never achieved sterilizing immunity (Bancroft *et al.*, 1986; Bhardwaj *et al.*, 1998). Examination at 6 h postinfection demonstrated equivalent numbers of bacteria in conventional versus immunocompromised strains of mice (Carrero *et al.*, 2006). In contrast, after 4 days of infection, SCID/*Rag*$^{-/-}$ mice harbored 100–1000-fold fewer *L. monocytogenes* than wild-type counterparts. The resistance phenotype was independent of input dose of infection as similar results were obtained after inoculation with a 10-fold range of bacteria. The resistance phenotype of SCID/*Rag*$^{-/-}$ was not due to increased number of preactivated macrophages: they did not show signs of activation prior to infection. Moreover, there was a significant reduction in the production of inflammatory cytokines during the first 4 days of infection in SCID/*Rag*$^{-/-}$ mice when compared to controls. As expected, examination of the spleens of SCID mice showed very few TUNEL^{+} cells following infection. Even after administering the type I IFN agonist poly(I:C), SCID mice did not develop increased leukocyte apoptosis following infection. Poly(I:C) did not cause increased growth of bacteria in SCID mice, despite a 10–100-fold increase in bacterial growth in wild-type counterparts (Carrero *et al.*, 2006). The results pointed to lymphocyte apoptosis as a component in the reduction of the innate resistance to *L. monocytogenes* infection *in vivo*: in their absence early resistance developed.

Reconstitution of the immunodeficient mice with bone marrow cells allowed us to establish the relationship between lymphocyte apoptosis and the early susceptibility to infection. *Rag2*$^{-/-}$ mice reconstituted with bone marrow became as susceptible to infection as normal mice: there was an increase in bacterial burden of approximately 1000-fold in *Rag2*$^{-/-}$ mice transplanted with wild-type bone marrow when compared to the controls (*Rag2*$^{-/-}$ mice and *Rag2*$^{-/-}$ mice transplanted with *Rag2*$^{-/-}$ bone marrow). This was clear proof that the presence of lymphocytes in the spleen contributed to the increased susceptibility to infection of normal mice compared to immunodeficient mice. Importantly, engraftment of IFN-αβR$^{-/-}$ bone marrow into *Rag2*$^{-/-}$ mice did not lead to increased susceptibility to infection. An additional condition was the engraftment of *Rag2*$^{-/-}$ mice with a 5 to 1 ratio of *Rag2*$^{-/-}$ to IFN-αβR$^{-/-}$ bone marrow. In this setting, all the lymphocytes developed from IFN-αβR$^{-/-}$ bone marrow progenitors, while all other leukocyte compartments developed from either *Rag2*$^{-/-}$ or IFN-αβR$^{-/-}$. We were able to screen the blood of chimeric mice and found a cohort that had 80–95% of the CD11b^{+} cells in circulation as IFN-αβR^{+} and >95% of the CD3^{+} cells as IFN-αβR^{-}. The mixed chimera mice were still resistant to infection with *L. monocytogenes*, indicating that type I interferon sensitivity by lymphocytes was required for increased susceptibility to infection. As mentioned previously, increased inflammatory cytokine production was found in mice that were more susceptible to infection. These studies on immunodeficient mice explained the heightened resistance of IFN-αβR$^{-/-}$ mice to infection. They established the role of lymphocyte apoptosis as a seminal component that modulated the resistance or susceptibility to infection.

7. CONCLUDING REMARKS

L. monocytogenes induces cell death in multiple immune and nonimmune cell types both *in vivo* and *in vitro*. The expression of LLO is required for the induction of cell death, and LLO can induce cell death as a purified protein. There is substantial evidence for the negative effect of cell death on the control of infection in mice. In almost all cases, more cell death correlates with increased susceptibility to infection. Of all the cell death pathways induced by *L. monocytogenes*, the lymphocyte apoptosis is the best understood. Future studies should examine the timing and mechanism of cell death in macrophage and dendritic cell subsets following infection.

We envision a scenario where the cell death process induced by *L. monocytogenes* weakens the innate immune response and possibly dampens adaptive immunity by causing nonspecific death of T cells.

It would be worthwhile to find mutations of LLO that do not lead to cell death but still permit escape of the pathogen to the cytosol. This would reinforce the claim that LLO is the direct apoptotic agent following infection. Since LLO-deficient bacteria are poorly immunogenic *in vivo*, having a strain that did not induce cell death, but still gained access to the cytosol, might permit generation of less virulent and more potent vaccine strains of *L. monocytogenes*.

The role of type I interferons on susceptibility to bacterial infections beside *L. monocytogenes* has been examined in a number of infections (Decker *et al.*, 2005; Trinchieri, 2010). In addition to the reports we have cited on the role of type I interferon in the EGD and 10403S strains of *L. monocytogenes*, there was also an association of increased virulence in a strain of *L. monocytogenes* that induced stronger type I interferon responses. The LO28 strain induced stronger type I interferon production and IRF-3 activation than the EGD strain and this correlated with an increased virulence following infection of mice (Reutterer *et al.*, 2008). The effect of type I interferon can be detrimental to mice following infection with other bacteria, such as *Francisella* spp., *Mycobacterium tuberculosis, Chlamydia muridarum*.

In the case of *Francisella*, IFN-αβR$^{-/-}$ mice were more resistant to infection due to an inhibitory effect of type I interferon signaling on IL-17 production (Henry and Monack, 2007). A separate report showed that *Francisella* induced extensive caspase-3 activation and apoptotic cell death in multiple tissues of infected mice (Wickstrum *et al.*, 2009). The possible association of type I interferon and apoptosis in *Francisella* remains unexplored.

In the case of *M. tuberculosis* infection, there was a survival benefit in infected IFN-αβR$^{-/-}$ mice (Manca *et al.*, 2005). There was also a correlation between susceptibility to infection and the ability of different strains of *M. tuberculosis* to induce type I interferon. As was found with *L. monocytogenes*, higher induction of type I interferon was associated with increased mortality following *M. tuberculosis* infection. *M. tuberculosis* induces the apoptosis of many immune cell types including T cells, but the relationship between type I interferon and apoptosis remains undefined.

IFN-αβR$^{-/-}$ mice were more resistant to a pulmonary infection with *C. muridarum* (Qiu *et al.*, 2008). Examination of lungs by immunofluorescence revealed caspase-3 activation that colocalized with the macrophage specific marker F4/80. The authors argued that the induction of macrophage death was, in part, responsible for the susceptibility to infection downstream of type I interferon signaling.

There are also bacterial species for which a type I interferon response is protective (i.e., *Salmonella typhimurium* and *Streptococcus pneumoniae*). It is still unclear why there are divergent effects of type I interferon signaling on different bacterial species (Trinchieri, 2010).

In sum, the robust lymphocyte apoptotic stage during *L. monocytogenes* infection with its important consequences has called attention to this phenomenon as playing a potential role in infections. In no other infectious disease studied at present is this stage so evident and the consequences so clear as in listeriosis. The degree to which apoptosis influences the outcome of different infections will depend on numerous variables. Many of these variables have been determined following *L. monocytogenes* infection and should serve as a guideline for future studies.

ACKNOWLEDGMENTS

Our thanks go to our colleague Boris Calderon who participated in a number of our studies. We would like to thank Sagar Chokshi for help in preparing the manuscript. The project described was supported by Grant Number AI062832 and MRCE U54 AI0571560, from the National Institute of Allergy and Infectious Disease (NIAID). Its contents are solely the responsibility of the authors and do not necessarily represent the official views of the NIAID or NIH.

REFERENCES

Aoshi, T., Carrero, J. A., Konjufca, V., Koide, Y., Unanue, E. R., and Miller, M. J. (2009). The cellular niche of *Listeria monocytogenes* infection changes rapidly in the spleen. *Eur. J. Immunol.* **39,** 417.

Auerbuch, V., Brockstedt, D. G., Meyer-Morse, N., O'Riordan, M., and Portnoy, D. A. (2004). Mice lacking the type I interferon receptor are resistant to *Listeria monocytogenes. J. Exp. Med.* **200,** 527.

Bancroft, G. J., Bosma, M. J., Bosma, G. C., and Unanue, E. R. (1986). Regulation of macrophage Ia expression in mice with severe combined immunodeficiency: Induction of Ia expression by a T cell-independent mechanism. *J. Immunol.* **137,** 4.

Barsig, J., and Kaufmann, S. H. (1997). The mechanism of cell death in *Listeria monocytogenes*-infected murine macrophages is distinct from apoptosis. *Infect. Immun.* **65,** 4075.

Bhardwaj, V., Kanagawa, O., Swanson, P. E., and Unanue, E. R. (1998). Chronic Listeria infection in SCID mice: Requirements for the carrier state and the dual role of T cells in transferring protection or suppression. *J. Immunol.* **160,** 376.

Bougnoux, P., Salem, N., Lyons, C., and Hoffman, T. (1985). Alteration in the membrane fatty acid composition of human lymphocytes and cultured transformed cells induced by interferon. *Mol. Immunol.* **22,** 1107.

Browne, K. A., Blink, E., Sutton, V. R., Froelich, C. J., Jans, D. A., and Trapani, J. A. (1999). Cytosolic delivery of granzyme B by bacterial toxins: Evidence that endosomal disruption, in addition to transmembrane pore formation, is an important function of perforin. *Mol. Cell. Biol.* **19,** 8604.

Carrero, J. A., and Unanue, E. R. (2006). Lymphocyte apoptosis as an immune subversion strategy of microbial pathogens. *Trends Immunol.* **27,** 497.

Carrero, J. A., Calderon, B., and Unanue, E. R. (2004a). Listeriolysin O from *Listeria monocytogenes* is a lymphocyte apoptogenic molecule. *J. Immunol.* **172,** 4866.

Carrero, J. A., Calderon, B., and Unanue, E. R. (2004b). Type I interferon sensitizes lymphocytes to apoptosis and reduces resistance to *Listeria* infection. *J. Exp. Med.* **200,** 535.

Carrero, J. A., Calderon, B., and Unanue, E. R. (2006). Lymphocytes are detrimental during the early innate immune response against Listeria monocytogenes. *J. Exp. Med.* **203,** 933.

Carrero, J. A., Vivanco-Cid, H., and Unanue, E. R. (2008). Granzymes drive a rapid listeriolysin O-induced T cell apoptosis. *J. Immunol.* **181,** 1365.

Carrero, J. A., Calderon, B., Vivanco-Cid, H., and Unanue, E. R. (2009). Recombinant Listeria monocytogenes expressing a cell wall-associated listeriolysin O is weakly virulent but immunogenic. *Infect. Immun.* **77,** 4371.

Cervantes, J., Nagata, T., Uchijima, M., Shibata, K., and Koide, Y. (2008). Intracytosolic *Listeria monocytogenes* induces cell death through caspase-1 activation in murine macrophages. *Cell. Microbiol.* **10,** 41.

Chan, Y. Y., and Cheers, C. (1982). Mechanism of depletion of T lymphocytes from the spleen of mice infected with *Listeria monocytogenes. Infect. Immun.* **38,** 686.

Chen, Q., Gong, B., Mahmoud-Ahmed, A. S., Zhou, A., Hsi, E. D., Hussein, M., and Almasan, A. (2001). Apo2L/TRAIL and Bcl-2-related proteins regulate type I interferon-induced apoptosis in multiple myeloma. *Blood* **98,** 2183.

Conlan, J. W., and North, R. J. (1994). Neutrophils are essential for early anti-*Listeria* defense in the liver, but not in the spleen or peritoneal cavity, as revealed by a granulocyte-depleting monoclonal antibody. *J. Exp. Med.* **179,** 259.

Dai, W. J., Kohler, G., and Brombacher, F. (1997). Both innate and acquired immunity to *Listeria monocytogenes* infection are increased in IL-10-deficient mice. *J. Immunol.* **158,** 2259.

Decker, T., Muller, M., and Stockinger, S. (2005). The yin and yang of type I interferon activity in bacterial infection. *Nat. Rev. Immunol.* **5,** 675.

Dresing, P., Borkens, S., Kocur, M., Kropp, S., and Scheu, S. (2010). A fluorescence reporter model defines "Tip-DCs" as the cellular source of interferon beta in murine listeriosis. *PLoS One* **5,** e15567.

Edelson, B. T., and Unanue, E. R. (2001). Intracellular antibody neutralizes *Listeria* growth. *Immunity* **14,** 503.

Edelson, B. T., Cossart, P., and Unanue, E. R. (1999). Cutting edge: Paradigm revisited: Antibody provides resistance to *Listeria* infection. *J. Immunol.* **163,** 4087.

Feng, H., Zhang, D., Palliser, D., Zhu, P., Cai, S., Schlesinger, A., Maliszewski, L., and Lieberman, J. (2005). *Listeria*-infected myeloid dendritic cells produce IFN-beta, priming T cell activation. *J. Immunol.* **175,** 421.

Gaillard, J. L., Berche, P., and Sansonetti, P. (1986). Transposon mutagenesis as a tool to study the role of hemolysin in the virulence of *Listeria monocytogenes. Infect. Immun.* **52,** 50.

Gilbert, R. J. (2010). Cholesterol-dependent cytolysins. *Adv. Exp. Med. Biol.* **677,** 56.

Glomski, I. J., Gedde, M. M., Tsang, A. W., Swanson, J. A., and Portnoy, D. A. (2002). The *Listeria monocytogenes* hemolysin has an acidic pH optimum to compartmentalize activity and prevent damage to infected host cells. *J. Cell Biol.* **156,** 1029.

Glomski, I. J., Decatur, A. L., and Portnoy, D. A. (2003). *Listeria monocytogenes* mutants that fail to compartmentalize listerolysin O activity are cytotoxic, avirulent, and unable to evade host extracellular defenses. *Infect. Immun.* **71,** 6754.

Guzman, C. A., Domann, E., Rohde, M., Bruder, D., Darji, A., Weiss, S., Wehland, J., Chakraborty, T., and Timmis, K. N. (1996). Apoptosis of mouse dendritic cells is triggered by listeriolysin, the major virulence determinant of *Listeria monocytogenes. Mol. Microbiol.* **20,** 119.

Henry, T., and Monack, D. M. (2007). Activation of the inflammasome upon Francisella tularensis infection: Interplay of innate immune pathways and virulence factors. *Cell. Microbiol.* **9,** 2543.

Heuck, A. P., Moe, P. C., and Johnson, B. B. (2010). The cholesterol-dependent cytolysin family of gram-positive bacterial toxins. *Subcell. Biochem.* **51,** 551.

Honda, K., Takaoka, A., and Taniguchi, T. (2006). Type I interferon gene induction by the interferon regulatory factor family of transcription factors. *Immunity* **25,** 349.

Jiang, J., Lau, L. L., and Shen, H. (2003). Selective depletion of nonspecific T cells during the early stage of immune responses to infection. *J. Immunol.* **171,** 4352.

Joseph, S. B., Bradley, M. N., Castrillo, A., Bruhn, K. W., Mak, P. A., Pei, L., Hogenesch, J., O'Connell, R. M., Cheng, G., Saez, E., Miller, J. F., and Tontonoz, P. (2004). LXR-dependent gene expression is important for macrophage survival and the innate immune response. *Cell* **119,** 299.

Kayal, S., and Charbit, A. (2006). Listeriolysin O: A key protein of *Listeria monocytogenes* with multiple functions. *FEMS Microbiol. Rev.* **30,** 514.

Manca, C., Tsenova, L., Freeman, S., Barczak, A. K., Tovey, M., Murray, P. J., Barry, C., and Kaplan, G. (2005). Hypervirulent M. tuberculosis W/Beijing strains upregulate type I IFNs and increase expression of negative regulators of the Jak-Stat pathway. *J. Interferon Cytokine Res.* **25,** 694.

Mandel, T. E., and Cheers, C. (1980). Resistance and susceptibility of mice to bacterial infection: Histopathology of listeriosis in resistant and susceptible strains. *Infect. Immun.* **30,** 851.

Masson, D., and Tschopp, J. (1987). A family of serine esterases in lytic granules of cytolytic T lymphocytes. *Cell* **49,** 679.

McCaffrey, R. L., Fawcett, P., O'Riordan, M., Lee, K. D., Havell, E. A., Brown, P. O., and Portnoy, D. A. (2004). A specific gene expression program triggered by Gram-positive bacteria in the cytosol. *Proc. Natl. Acad. Sci. USA* **101,** 11386.

Merrick, J. C., Edelson, B. T., Bhardwaj, V., Swanson, P. E., and Unanue, E. R. (1997). Lymphocyte apoptosis during early phase of *Listeria* infection in mice. *Am. J. Pathol.* **151,** 785.

Muraille, E., Giannino, R., Guirnalda, P., Leiner, I., Jung, S., Pamer, E. G., and Lauvau, G. (2005). Distinct in vivo dendritic cell activation by live versus killed *Listeria monocytogenes*. *Eur. J. Immunol.* **35,** 1463.

Neuenhahn, M., Kerksiek, K. M., Nauerth, M., Suhre, M. H., Schiemann, M., Gebhardt, F. E., Stemberger, C., Panthel, K., Schroder, S., Chakraborty, T., Jung, S., Hochrein, H., *et al.* (2006). CD8alpha + dendritic cells are required for efficient entry of *Listeria monocytogenes* into the spleen. *Immunity* **25,** 619.

O'Connell, R. M., Saha, S. K., Vaidya, S. A., Bruhn, K. W., Miranda, G. A., Zarnegar, B., Perry, A. K., Nguyen, B. O., Lane, T. F., Taniguchi, T., Miller, J. F., and Cheng, G. (2004). Type I interferon production enhances susceptibility to *Listeria monocytogenes* infection. *J. Exp. Med.* **200,** 437.

O'Riordan, M., Yi, C. H., Gonzales, R., Lee, K. D., and Portnoy, D. A. (2002). Innate recognition of bacteria by a macrophage cytosolic surveillance pathway. *Proc. Natl. Acad. Sci. USA* **99,** 13861.

Portnoy, D. A., Jacks, P. S., and Hinrichs, D. J. (1988). Role of hemolysin for the intracellular growth of *Listeria monocytogenes*. *J. Exp. Med.* **167,** 1459.

Qiu, H., Fan, Y., Joyee, A. G., Wang, S., Han, X., Bai, H., Jiao, L., Van Rooijen, N., and Yang, X. (2008). Type I IFNs enhance susceptibility to *Chlamydia muridarum* lung infection by enhancing apoptosis of local macrophages. *J. Immunol.* **181,** 2092.

Reutterer, B., Stockinger, S., Pilz, A., Soulat, D., Kastner, R., Westermayer, S., Rulicke, T., Muller, M., and Decker, T. (2008). Type I IFN are host modulators of strain-specific *Listeria monocytogenes* virulence. *Cell. Microbiol.* **10,** 1116.

Rogers, H. W., and Unanue, E. R. (1993). Neutrophils are involved in acute, nonspecific resistance to *Listeria monocytogenes* in mice. *Infect. Immun.* **61,** 5090.

Rogers, H. W., Callery, M. P., Deck, B., and Unanue, E. R. (1996). *Listeria monocytogenes* induces apoptosis of infected hepatocytes. *J. Immunol.* **156,** 679.

Rosado, C. J., Buckle, A. M., Law, R. H., Butcher, R. E., Kan, W. T., Bird, C. H., Ung, K., Browne, K. A., Baran, K., Bashtannyk-Puhalovich, T. A., Faux, N. G., Wong, W., *et al.* (2007). A common fold mediates vertebrate defense and bacterial attack. *Science* **317,** 1548.

Sauer, J. D., Witte, C. E., Zemansky, J., Hanson, B., Lauer, P., and Portnoy, D. A. (2010). Listeria monocytogenes triggers AIM2-mediated pyroptosis upon infrequent bacteriolysis in the macrophage cytosol. *Cell Host Microbe* **7,** 412.

Schluter, D., Domann, E., Buck, C., Hain, T., Hof, H., Chakraborty, T., and Deckert-Schluter, M. (1998). Phosphatidylcholine-specific phospholipase C from Listeria monocytogenes is an important virulence factor in murine cerebral listeriosis. *Infect. Immun.* **66,** 5930.

Schnupf, P., and Portnoy, D. A. (2007). Listeriolysin O: A phagosome-specific lysin. *Microbes Infect.* **9,** 1176.

Singh, R., Jamieson, A., and Cresswell, P. (2008). GILT is a critical host factor for *Listeria monocytogenes* infection. *Nature* **455,** 1244.

Stockinger, S., Kastner, R., Kernbauer, E., Pilz, A., Westermayer, S., Reutterer, B., Soulat, D., Stengl, G., Vogl, C., Frenz, T., Waibler, Z., Taniguchi, T., *et al.* (2009). Characterization of the interferon-producing cell in mice infected with *Listeria monocytogenes. PLoS Pathog.* **5,** e1000355.

Sun, S., Zhang, X., Tough, D. F., and Sprent, J. (1998). Type I interferon-mediated stimulation of T cells by CpG DNA. *J. Exp. Med.* **188,** 2335.

Tang, P., Rosenshine, I., Cossart, P., and Finlay, B. B. (1996). Listeriolysin O activates mitogen-activated protein kinase in eucaryotic cells. *Infect. Immun.* **64,** 2359.

Trinchieri, G. (2010). Type I interferon: Friend or foe? *J. Exp. Med.* **207,** 2053.

Wadsworth, S. J., and Goldfine, H. (1999). *Listeria monocytogenes* phospholipase C-dependent calcium signaling modulates bacterial entry into J774 macrophage-like cells. *Infect. Immun.* **67,** 1770.

Wickstrum, J. R., Bokhari, S. M., Fischer, J. L., Pinson, D. M., Yeh, H. W., Horvat, R. T., and Parmely, M. J. (2009). Francisella tularensis induces extensive caspase-3 activation and apoptotic cell death in the tissues of infected mice. *Infect. Immun.* **77,** 4827.

Zheng, S. J., Jiang, J., Shen, H., and Chen, Y. H. (2004). Reduced apoptosis and ameliorated listeriosis in TRAIL-null mice. *J. Immunol.* **173,** 5652.

Zwaferink, H., Stockinger, S., Hazemi, P., Lemmens-Gruber, R., and Decker, T. (2008). IFN-beta increases listeriolysin O-induced membrane permeabilization and death of macrophages. *J. Immunol.* **180,** 4116.

INDEX

D

M

N

P

CONTENTS OF RECENT VOLUMES

Volume 88

Volume 89

Volume 90

Volume 91

Volume 92

Volume 93

Volume 94

Volume 95

Volume 96

Volume 97

Volume 98

Volume 99

Volume 100

Volume 101

Volume 102

Volume 103

Volume 104

Volume 105

Volume 106

Volume 107

Volume 108

Volume 109

Volume 110

Volume 111

Volume 112

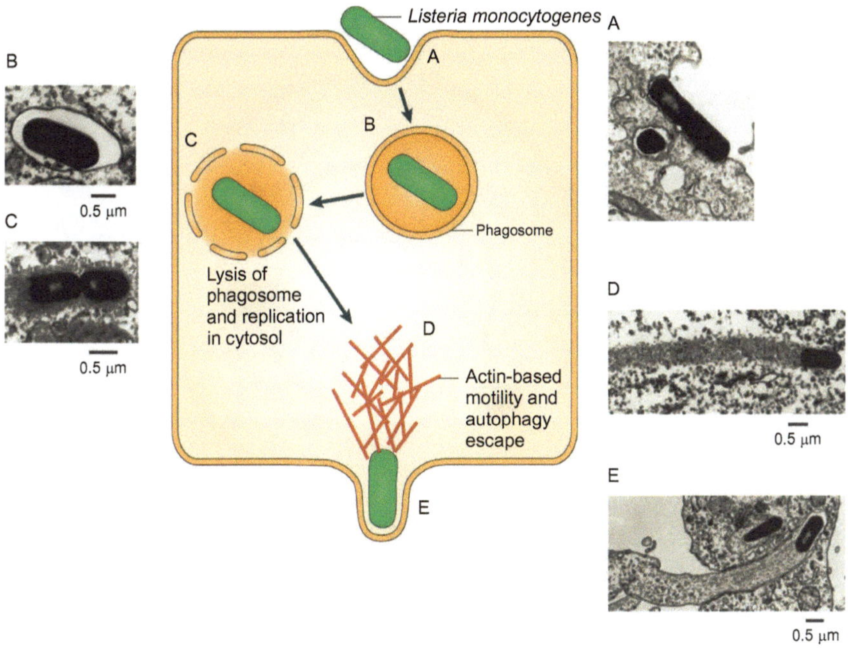

Chapter 3, Figure 3.1 (See page 21 of this volume.)

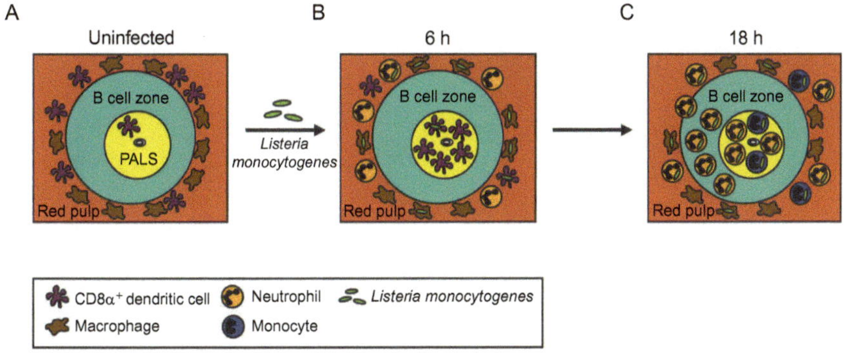

Chapter 4, Figure 4.1 (See page 40 of this volume.)

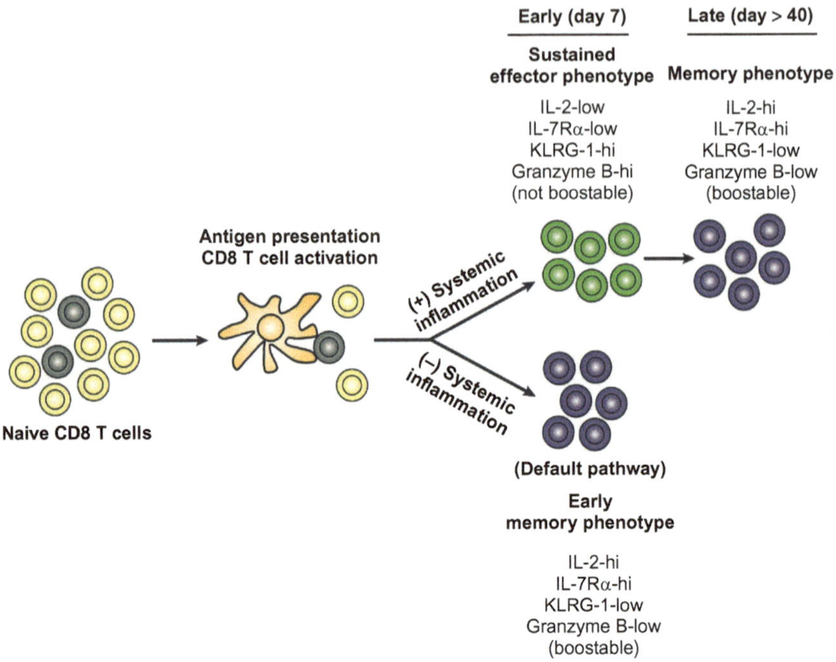

Chapter 5, Figure 5.2 (See page 64 of this volume.)

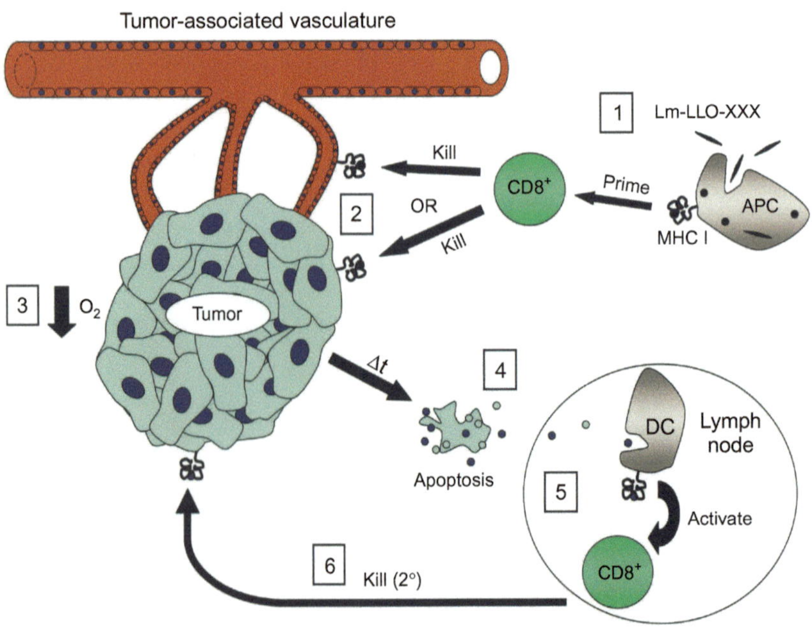

Chapter 6, Figure 6.3 (See page 100 of this volume.)

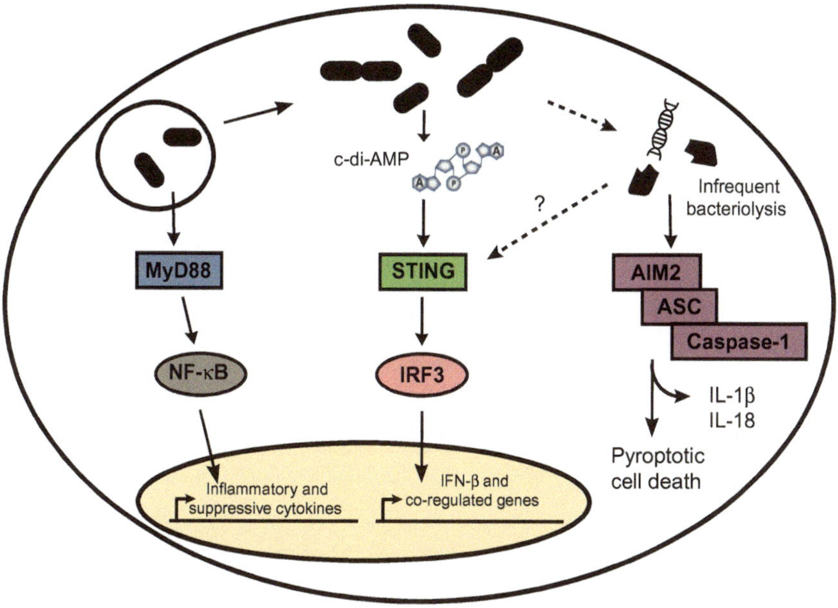

Chapter 8, Figure 8.1 **(See page 138 of this volume.)**

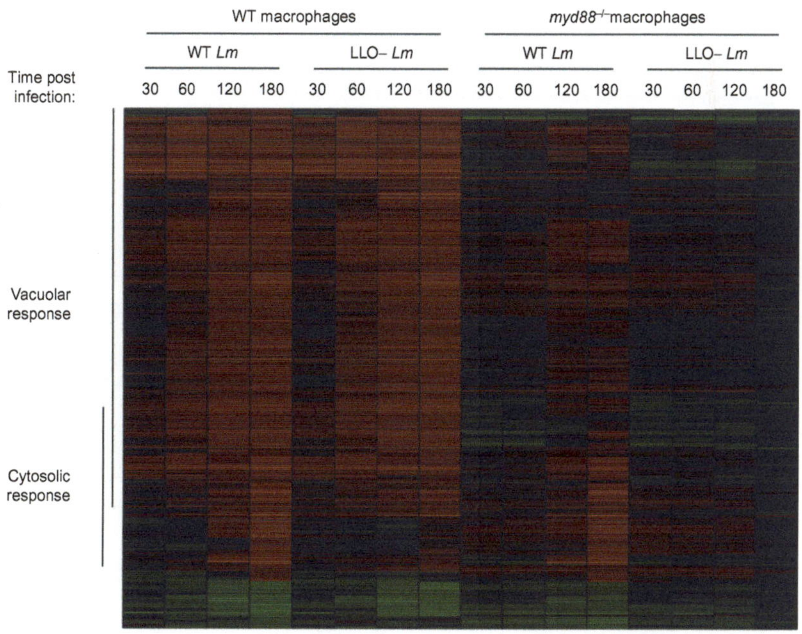

Chapter 8, Figure 8.2 **(See page 140 of this volume.)**

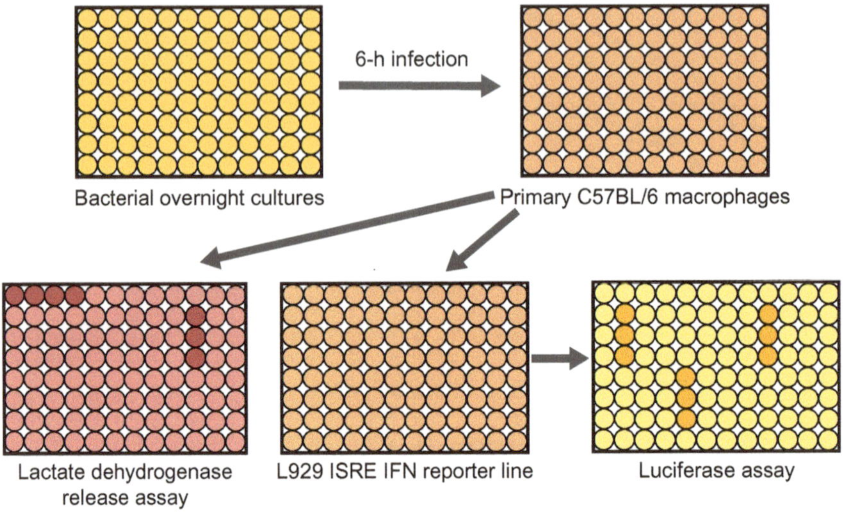

Chapter 8, Figure 8.3 **(See page 142 of this volume.)**

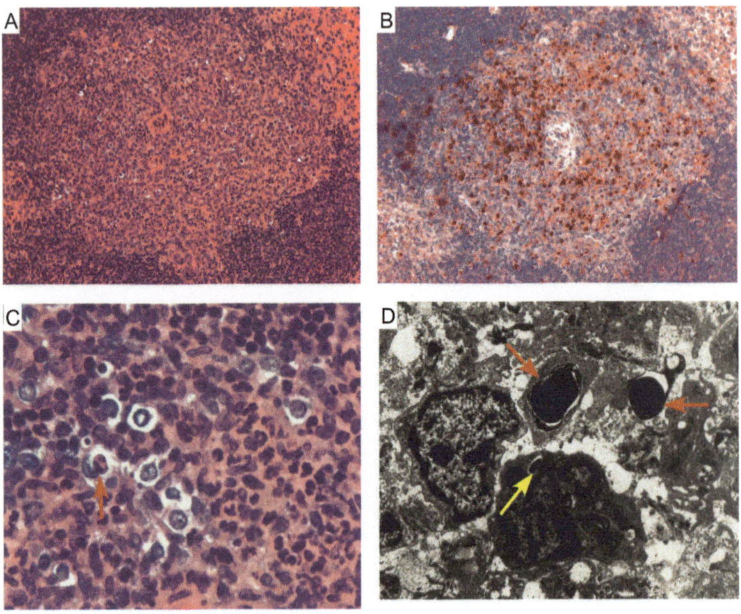

Chapter 9, Figure 9.1 **(See page 159 of this volume.)**

FSC
www.fsc.org
MIX
Papier | Fördert
gute Waldnutzung
FSC® C083411

Kolibri 360 GmbH
Ferdinand-Jühlke-Straße 7
99095 Erfurt, Deutschland
produktsicherheit@kolibri360.de